G000271398

This series introduces a wide range of healing techniques that can be used either independently or as a complement to traditional medical treatment. Most of the techniques included in the series can be learnt and practised alone, and each encourages a degree of self-reliance, offering the tools needed to achieve and maintain an optimum state of health.

Each title opens with information on the history and principles of the technique and goes on to offer practical and straightforward guidance on ways in which it can be applied, with diagrams and case studies where appropriate. Please note that readers are advised to seek professional guidance for serious ailments, and to make use of the list of practitioners for further guidance. Many of the techniques in this series are taught in workshops and adult education classes; all of the titles are written by professional practitioners with many years of experience and proven track records.

AVAILABLE IN THIS SERIES

Healing with Colour — Helen Graham

Healing with Homeopathy — Peter Chappell and
   David Andrews

Healing with Meditation — Doriel Hall

Healing with Osteopathy — Peta Sneddon and Paolo Coseschi

Healing with Reflexology — Rosalind Oxenford

FORTHCOMING TITLES IN THIS SERIES

Healing with Ayurveda

Healing with Chinese Medicine

Healing with Crystals

Healing with Essential Oils

Healing with Feng Shui

Healing with Flower Essences

Healing with Nutritional Therapy

Healing with Shiatsu

Healing with Herbs

JUDITH HOAD

Gill & Macmillan

Gill & Macmillan Ltd
Goldenbridge
Dublin 8
with associated companies throughout the world
© Judith Hoad 1996
0 7171 2454 1
Series editor: Tessa Strickland
Series copy editor: Pamela Dix
Index compiled by Helen Litton
Print origination by Typeform Repro Ltd, Dublin
Printed by ColourBooks Ltd, Dublin

A catalogue record is available for this book from the
British Library.

1   3   5   4   2

Contents

CHAPTER ONE

Why Herbal Remedies?

Plant life has been used as food and as medication for as long as we know. In China and in India, herbal medicine has a continuous history going back thousands of years. The Chinese still use a medical text that dates to six hundred years before the birth of Jesus. Indian medicine, known as Ayurveda, refers to texts that are even older. We can therefore infer that the medical practices to which these works refer were in existence for many — perhaps hundreds — of years before the books were written.

HERBAL MEDICINE AND NATURE

Herbal medicine, by being an integral part of nature, in itself an integral part of human life — in so far as we allow it to be — is accessible to anyone who wishes to use it. There have been notable experts down the ages who have practised and taught about herbal medicine. By its very accessibility and openness to local tradition, however, it has also been practised by many thousands of lay practitioners, the majority of whom have been women.

I have not written this book for experts or for trained herbalists, but for that continuum of lay practitioners, of whom I have been one for the last thirty years. As I have been writing, I have deliberately concentrated on the disorders that most people encounter from time to time, things commonplace rather than rare. Not all the herbs that help these problems are listed, but the most common ones are. The plants are easily found in the appropriate habitat,

and they are easily grown as well. Sources of seed for those
who wish to grow their own healing herbs are listed in
'Helpful Addresses', pages 117–18.

I hope that exploring the plant life around the fields,
city parks, cottage gardens or window-boxes amongst
which you live will enrich your life, as it has enriched
mine. Herbalism, lay or professional, is a nature-related
practice that can only serve to bring us to a better
awareness of our relationship with all life around us, and
turn us away from the destructiveness of the 'gimme'
society that western consumerism has created.

THE FAILURE OF ORTHODOX MEDICINE

As more and more people experience the inadequacies of
orthodox, allopathic medicine, having to endure
sometimes misery-making side-effects from treatment, so
more and more are driven by desperation to find some
other, personally predictable, way to cope with accidents
and disease. Some people are also seeking a more positive
way to approach health maintenance and the treatment of
disorder. For these people, it is not so much their
experiences of using orthodox medicine as the philosophy
behind it that puts them off.

Our entire culture is obsessed with quantitative
materialism and with technological advances in all
directions — a technology that is based on the explosive
principle, never on the implosive. Orthodox medical
practices, reflecting mainstream culture and the analytical
techniques endemic in quantitative materialism, have
reduced the individual from the reality of an amalgam of
inseparable parts that can be grouped and spoken about
under four headings, physical, emotional, mental and
spiritual — but which cannot be separated — to a 'case' of

whatever seems to be the trouble at the time. The treatment offered by the orthodoxy will be one designed to kill the invading bacterium, virus, cancer cell, or whatever it is. Herbal medicine, on the other hand, uses creatures full of natural energy (plants), working to restore the life energy of the individual, often on all the levels mentioned above, or at least on more than one of them.

HERBAL MEDICINE AS SELF-EMPOWERMENT

In its accessibility, herbal medicine can be adopted as an aspect of self-empowerment. This is not to use the term self-empowerment as it is usually used — to describe a politically assertive condition. In this context, I am using the term to describe exactly the power we take that gives us the ability to respond — and thereby take '*respons-ibility*' — to situations that arise in our lives. Some of these situations will inevitably concern our individual health and health maintenance.

Health maintenance is not a conscious concern of the majority of people. Mostly, it is only when we experience the breakdown of our health that we respond by taking steps to readjust to good health. However, it is often the 'discovery' of herbal medicine, or another of the so-called alternative medical practices, that leads the individual to find many more unorthodox ways to sustain a healthy life, and to do what we all should aspire to: live life to the fullest potential that our body and mind can enable us.

The practice of a broad-based, home-administered, herbalism can assure every member of the household a continuous sense of well-being. Seasonal dishes from seasonal growths of wild and cultivated plants — especially those that know no chemical additives in their growth or cultivation — will give health and energy to each person

eating them, something that is impossible to find in the
fast-food, instant-satisfaction ethos of the late twentieth
century. Fast food is for people who don't respect their
bodily systems, nor understand the virtues of the titillatory
anticipation created by the smells of cooking. Nor can
they enjoy, because they've never tried it, the slow
mastication that extracts the varied tastes of wholesome,
organic, unprocessed foods. Fast food is for those who
eventually develop ulcers in the stomach, or the
duodenum, or the colon, and then expect an equally
quick-fix medicine which will put them right, while
allowing them to continue eating fast food, fast.

THE CONFIDENCE BARRIER

This book is for people who want to slow down, for those
who can acknowledge that we all have choices — it is
only our lack of imagination that blinds us to them. For
this reason, I am going to deal with the confidence barrier,
and share with you case histories that may encourage you
to the self-empowered leap over that barrier (see 'Case
Studies', pages 111–16). Breaking the confidence barrier is
the first step to becoming your own physician.

DIAGNOSIS

All healing techniques depend for their success on accurate
diagnosis. This book is not a guide to diagnosis. If you are
in doubt about what is wrong, an orthodox general
practitioner is usually dependable and you should therefore
contact your own GP. Describe to her or him the
symptoms and signs of which you are aware. It helps to
write these down as a list before you telephone, or before
you make a visit to the doctor's surgery. Be as brief and as
accurate as possible. For example, if you are describing pain

— your own, or someone else's — use adjectives such as 'dull', 'stabbing', 'burning', 'recurrent' or 'intermittent'; show the area of the pain by saying whether you can cover it with your fingertip, the palm of your hand, or whatever is applicable. Remember, of course, to say where the pain is in the body.

State whether there is fever, or not. If you do not have a thermometer, you will find that the brow and temples of a person with fever will be hot to the touch. Their tongue will also probably be reddish; any 'fur', or 'moss', on it will be yellowish. Their pulse rate may be increased as well. This can be judged by finding the radial artery in the wrist and watching the person's breathing pattern. If they have more than four pulse beats to one cycle of inhalation and exhalation, then they probably have a fever, especially if some or all of the other signs I have mentioned are also present. If you are talking to the doctor on the telephone, this information will be invaluable in helping him or her to come to a diagnosis.

If the doctor offers you a prescription, it may be diplomatic to accept it — it's only a piece of paper. You are not obliged to have it made up, nor to take it. If you decide not to have it made up, destroy it. This action is part of dismantling the confidence barrier.

RESCUE REMEDY AND FIVE FLOWER REMEDY

Plants are not always used in their material form. Throughout this book I refer to Rescue Remedy and Five Flower Remedy. They are the same thing, but named differently by the two firms that make them. They both come directly from the philosophy and research of an orthodox doctor, Dr Edward Bach, a man of great

eminence, after whom a technique in renal surgery is
named and still used.

Dr Bach gave up his orthodox practice in Harley
Street, London to devote the last years of his life to the
research and development of a range of thirty-eight
essences made from the flowers of plants and trees. Rescue
Remedy is the only combination of these flowers made by
the suppliers. Other combinations are the choice of the
individual, or their practitioner. Five Flower Remedy is
made by Julian and Martine Barnard in rural England, and
Rescue Remedy is made and supplied by Nelson's, the
homeopathic pharmacy.

Five Flower Remedy and Rescue Remedy, both —
unlike any of the other flower remedies — also available as
a cream, are remarkably efficient removers of shock in the
event of an accident, physical, or emotional, in any of the
situations that make the adrenalin run and instil the 'fight
or flight' reaction. The remedy removes the shock and
allows the body to resume its own repair work. The worse
the situation, the more dramatically the remedy works.
Lives are claimed to have been saved by it and in my
opinion no home should be without it. I carry mine with
me at all times and it is surprising how frequently it is
needed.

Flower essences are different from the results of the
other recipes, because they are closer to a homeopathic
preparation. Also, they are used from a broader basis than
non-homeopathic herbal remedies, for emotional, mental
and spiritual conditions out of which the physical
manifestation may, or may not, arise. What distinguishes
flower remedies from other herbal preparations is that they
are not individually indicated for specific physical
disorders. In fact, two individuals who, apparently, are

manifesting the same disorder at the physical level, may each need a totally different selection of flower remedies.

'INTENTION'

Using herbs, in whatever form — having first identified and harvested them — is a pathway to a new and fuller understanding of ourselves and the environment of which we are a part. In the process of re-learning what used to be common knowledge, I have found my experiences with plants enriched by incorporating an 'intention' in all my interactions with plants at every stage.

The intention is one that permeated every aspect of the lives of the native peoples of North and South America. They used rituals that honoured the plant source. They used — some still do — requests, gratitude and the sort of respect usually reserved in our society for an equal, as they harvested, processed and administered their remedies. I have no idea what their rituals were, but I use their intention. I find when I do this that I am incapable of exploiting the plants. I can only think of them and behave toward them as I would toward any respected neighbour or friend. This is something I have had to learn — I didn't inherit it from our European culture. It has enriched my life, and I hope it will enrich yours when you try it.

THE CONTEXT IN WHICH WE LIVE

In my experience, no book on herbal medicine contains the accurate illustrations found in botanical books designed for identifying wild plants. But on the other hand, the botanical books do not describe the medicinal uses of the plants shown. So whenever I am asked how I distinguish one plant from another, I show the botanical

book I use, in which there is nothing about herbal
medicine. It does, however, contain plenty of good
illustrations, with brief descriptions of the appearance,
habitat and flowering time of every plant.

This botanical handbook is about the wild plants of
the British Isles and Northern Europe, so I know I'm not
going to find anything in it about plants that grow in
distant countries. This, for me, is important, because I
believe we are better served by what grows around us than
by unfamiliar plants from faraway places. We and the
plants, insects, birds and animals that live in the same area
are in context with one another. In addition, we can
gather plants that grow around us with ease, and know
that they are collected, preserved and stored correctly.

Context is very important. I don't just believe it — it
makes itself obvious. For example, not long after starting to
read a book about herbal medicine, you will notice that
there are many different plants that have a very similar
virtue (or 'benefit to users', if you prefer). By consulting a
book of plant identification, one difference between plants
of similar virtue is shown to be habitat. Limey, or sandy, or
peaty soil preference, open or shaded areas, preferred
altitude and some or several perhaps will have a preference
for growing in a soil and at an altitude that is the same as
the one in which *you* live.

Have you ever thought how different your life would
have been if you had lived the last, say, ten years in a
different kind of house, on a different street, or on a
different hill, in a different town, in a different county —
or even on another continent? Your neighbours would
have been different, your job opportunities different, your
language, even, might have been different. Far more than
we realise, our environment of house, landscape — or

townscape — local community, weather conditions, geological base, colleagues and neighbours help to shape us to the people we have grown to be at any given time in our lives.

If I had continued to live in a city instead of moving to an isolated country area in 1967, I might still be a chain-smoking coffee addict. If I hadn't had teeth growing sideways and in the middle of my palate, I might not have discovered at the age of fifteen that I was allergic to penicillin, injected into me to prevent infection when I had five of the offending teeth surgically removed. Without the stress of city life I was able to give up the cigarettes and coffee and begin to discover the amazing variety of plants that grew in the fields and hedgerows around my new home. Penicillin gave me a severe outbreak of nettle rash — so itchy — and a permanent photosensitivity to ultra-violet light. The latter means that after a good dose of sunshine the rash starts up again, even now, forty-three years later.

The combination of the dental surgery at fifteen and the move to the country fifteen years later gave me the opportunity to explore plants that I could use for medicine rather than go to the doctor for drugs that made me worse rather than better. I had by then discovered other antibiotics to which I was allergic and that I am allergic to the anti-allergic drug, antihistamine! The frustration that this evoked in some doctors only accentuated for me the need to learn enough to be my own medicine finder. I had young children by then, too, and that also urged me on, because I didn't want them to have the same painful experiences I had had.

So, context means that if you live, for example, in an area of chalky soil, the water you drink will be what is

described as 'hard'. It will take a lot of soap to raise a
lather and the kettle will rapidly become coated with a
limey deposit from all the calcium that will precipitate
when the water boils. You will be more likely to have
strong bones, and be surrounded by lime-loving plants.
There will be roach and trout in the clear waters of the
local rivers and the land will drain easily. Farmers will
grow acres of grain and milk cows will be big and high-
yielding.

Conversely, if you live in a peaty area, on what is
referred to as 'acid' soil, the rivers will probably have water
the colour of bitter beer, soft and easy to lather. There will
be very little grain grown and places liable to flooding in
soil that retains water. Instead of the beeches and chestnuts
of the limey soils, pine, willows and poplars will grow.
There will be more grazing for meat and less for milk.

What grows around us is accessible and is in sympathy
with us because it too experiences the same weather and
environmental conditions that we do. If our environment
is heavily polluted, so will we and the plants around us be
— in fact, few healthy plants will grow in a heavily
polluted area. If you are unfortunate enough to live in this
sort of area, you will have to travel to find plants growing
in a healthy environment.

WESTERN CIVILISATION AND AGGRESSION

Pollution is an ever-present reminder that we are
challenged at the end of the twentieth century by the
misuse of our planet. The dominator tribes — usually
referred to as western civilisation — have taken an
aggressive, exploitative stance in all they have done. Much
of our language uses military terminology: we talk about
shooting pictures; *fortifying* the body; *fighting* disease;

conquering Tuberculosis, or Cancer, or AIDS. We use specific terms to classify people, governments, behaviour patterns, age groups and things we do not value. By this technique, unless a plant is being grown for profit, we regard it as a 'weed', which allows us at best to ignore it, at worst to destroy it. Yet that 'weed' is only a plant growing in the place of its own choosing — a volunteer, as you might say.

While we have punitive laws to discourage us from homicide, matricide, infanticide and so on, most farmers think nothing of surrounding — even drenching — the plants they grow for profit in insecticide, fungicide or herbicide. Cultivated plants, therefore, grow up saturated in an environment of death and killing.

In the wild state, plants grow in colonies, often interspersed with other species of plants that in some way will support or protect one another. In the days of permanent pasture, there were fields that were never ploughed, full of plants as well as grass. Those fields were mown to make hay for winter fodder and before the hay shed was filled with the fresh crop of hay, the floor was swept and the seed thus garnered was sown back on the freshly mown pasture fields so that a state of constant, annual renewal took place. The animals that grazed those pastures had the benefit of a multiplicity of plants that nourished them in a variety of ways, keeping them healthy and their milk and meat, hides and wool wholesome.

'LET YOUR MEDICINE BE YOUR FOOD AND YOUR FOOD BE YOUR MEDICINE'

When an orthodox, western doctor qualifies, he or she takes an oath, the origin of which is attributed to Hippocrates, a philosopher of Ancient Greece. The oath is

one in which the doctor promises to protect the lives of
his or her patients at all times. However, the same doctors
pay scant attention to something else attributed to
Hippocrates: the statement that we should 'let our
medicine be our food and our food be our medicine'. Can
you imagine a McDonald's burger being recommended for
your head cold? But a mixed salad of a variety of plants
growing round your garden, or a soup made from nettles
and nutmeg, either washed down with a cup of hot
elderflower tea, and you're well on the way to recovery!

By seeking out 'weeds' in our gardens, lanes, building
sites and hedgerows, we can become acquainted with our
environment and learn that these plants have virtues and
great variety, that they can help us, heal us and teach us
love for them and the places in which they grow. In fact,
they can re-connect us with our context and help us to
feel the way they and we belong where we are. Ironically,
many of today's 'weeds' are yesterday's cultivated crops:
Dandelion, Fat Hen, Lamb's Tongue Sorrel, Tansy and
many others were all under cultivation in and beyond
Elizabethan times.

SPECIALISATION AND DIVISIONS

Identifying and contextualising plants growing around us is
one thing, but finding a chink in the confidence barrier I
have talked about is quite another. Our dominator culture
has divided society into classes, stratified by income or
wealth, by professions and trades. Each division specialises
in one or another form of expertise, each tending to
isolate us from other divisions and each specialisation
acting to remove from us the power to respond to our
own needs. For example, few people design and build their
own houses. An architect, whose design is interpreted by a

builder, will do that for you, or if not for you personally, then for the housing association, or the council where you live.

If anything goes wrong with our health, we hand over responsibility to our GP, who may in turn hand over that responsibility by sending you to see a 'specialist', or a 'consultant' in a distant hospital. Many people complain that such highly qualified body-carers don't listen to them, the body-users, or take what they experience seriously. Or they ignore the sick person's desire to know about the medication they prescribe, what it's supposed to change in the body and if it is likely to have any 'side-effects' (the euphemism for allergic reaction) and what these might be. Most of us accept this as how it has to be. Yet it *does not* have to be this way.

Individually, we are each the world expert on our *own* bodies. No one else can know the sensation of our feelings, whether these are physical or emotional. If we take ourselves seriously, we can deal with most of the disorders we encounter without even informing the doctor. Thus, when an emergency crops up that we know we can't handle, our independent experiences can enable us to understand better what is offered by a doctor when we have called on her, or him.

Sometimes a single incident can take us through the confidence barrier; a time when there is no doctor to whom we can 'surrender' ourselves for treatment. For example, one day recently I was talking to a group of adults on a camping holiday about becoming your own herbalist when we heard a child start screaming while a dog barked. Maggie leapt up and dashed out of sight, having recognised both screamer and barker. Her son, aged six, had been bitten by the dog, who had been left on a

long tether in the hot sun with no access to shade.
Enraged by the usually welcome attentions of the little
boy, it had sunk its teeth into his arm.

'What shall I do?' asked Maggie. She had Hydrogen
Peroxide, the best disinfectant; she had Rescue Remedy
(see pages 5–6 for further information on these remedies)
the best anti-shock treatment; she had a little boy who had
faith in her because she was Mummy and there was no
doctor for miles. The Hydrogen Peroxide fizzed and
bubbled as it oxygenated the germs. The Rescue Remedy
calmed Charlie and let his body come out of shock to get
on with the repair work and Maggie chewed the Wound-
Wort that one of the group had picked from an unkempt
herbaceous border in the garden in which we were sitting.
She applied the Wound-Wort after the Peroxide had
worked for about ten minutes. The action Maggie took
was immediate and the result was a clean, neat wound that
healed very quickly. Next time there is a straightforward
medical emergency in her family, Maggie will be
confident to deal with it.

FIRST AID BOX

In order to deal with a situation requiring treatment, the
first necessity is a simple and readily accessible First Aid
Box. In mine I keep a few tools:

- scissors
- tweezers
- wooden tooth-picks (cocktail sticks answer the
  same need)
- safety pins
- adjustable dressings.

By adjustable dressings, I mean a roll of lint, two different
widths of crepe bandage and a packet of elasticated plaster

strip with dressing in the middle, from which the required width can be cut when needed.

A range of frequently updated herbal remedies and both cream and fluid Rescue Remedy or Five Flower Remedy completes the box.

Your First Aid Box should be portable, but your Medicine Chest or Emergency Store does not need to be. The Medicine Chest should contain:

- cotton or linen bedding (if not normally used in your house)
- woollen blankets
- plastic sheeting
- a bed pan or potty
- a thermometer
- clean cotton rags for poultices or compresses
- paper and cloth handkerchiefs.

A calibrated glass measure and your stored medicinal supplies — herbal and otherwise — can be kept in the Emergency Store, or wherever you find convenient.

Be aware that if homeopathic remedies — and in this instance, I would include flower essences such as Five Flower or Rescue Remedy — are among your stores, you should not place them near your herbal preparations or any other strong smelling substances like essential oils; this is because they will probably become nullified by such things.

Following treatment, I have found a record book a tremendous help. I write each step out in brief, as soon as possible, how I treated the problem and what the outcome was. This record has proved invaluable on many occasions.

CHAPTER TWO

The Origins of Herbal Medicine

THE BEGINNINGS

Herbal healing is necessary only if we become ill and the appropriate use of herbs can keep us in good health, preventing any illness from developing. This was the way in which humankind lived for millennia. By taking note of where certain plants or animals lived and thrived — or, conversely, the places that they shunned — humankind learned empirically about favourable and adverse energies. Sleeping places, birthing places, bleeding places, hunting and sowing and harvesting places were all found by a complex interaction of intuition and observation.

By allowing the spirit to wander, because like the mind it is a part of the human system able to do so, knowledge was shared with all other living creatures. Thus for millennia, plants and animals, both wild and domesticated, were mutually interdependent with people for all they needed in sickness and in health.

This interdependence is being destroyed in many regions of the world. For example, ecologists and Green activists are publicising the loss of potential medicinal plants as the rain forest of South America is reduced by wanton felling. Yet every domestic garden and rural hedgerow represents a miniature source of medicinal plants. Our own 'rain forest' is being destroyed on our very own doorsteps and no one is protesting about it. The difference is that the understanding and use of our native plants is neglected in preference to the exotic from far away.

Incidentally, the indigenous peoples of the Americas always considered the effect of their actions on the following seven generations, whether they were felling a tree or planting a garden — something we of the 'over-developed' parts of the world should emulate. For this reason, the rain forest survived until European exploiters arrived to destroy it for short-term grazing, after which the soil is no longer capable of re-establishing and sustaining the multi-level forest that once was home to plants, insects, reptiles, birds, animals and people.

TRADITIONAL CHINESE MEDICINE

Traditional Chinese medicine may be a little younger than the Ayurveda of India, although both have a medicinal history going back around 3,000 years. Chinese medicine has become fairly familiar in parts of the west, but Ayurveda is still somewhat obscure. Like the Chinese, the Indian tradition still uses texts — in their case Hindu scriptural texts — that date to the earliest times of their recorded history. Herbs figure centrally in both traditions.

THE NATURE OF *QI*

No form of medicine is in isolation from the common philosophy of the people who practise and use it. Chinese philosophy synthesises phenomena and recognises energy as a component in the balance that synthesis seeks to achieve. The word the Chinese use for energy is *qi,* sometimes spelled *chi,* and pronounced 'chee'. (Is it too obscure to suggest a possible connection between *qi* and the Irish word for the spirits of the plants, the *sidhe,* pronounced 'shee'?) *Qi* is a word that is gaining acceptance and use among unorthodox medical practitioners in the west, most of whom work with energy in some form.

Traditional Chinese medical practitioners, using the process of synthesis to diagnose and to treat their clients, do not use herbs in isolation. The tools and disciplines employed in addition to herbs include acupuncture, or acupressure, both techniques that access and can in a very direct way stimulate or sedate energy that is out of balance; moxibustion, dried Mugwort, burned, is another process for stimulating the energy in the body; through exercise forms called *qi gong*, the client can access the points of energy in the body after being taught the technique appropriate to the individual's imbalance; diet and meditation; massage.

Qi is a word that is used for many aspects of energy and there is more than one kind of *qi* in the body. The *qi* that is accessed in acupuncture or acupressure flows in distinct pathways over the torso, limbs and head. Only in the last twenty years or so have electronic tools been invented that are subtle enough to identify the points used on these pathways as areas of lowered electrical resistance. In Chinese medicine, herbs and diet would be prescribed bearing in mind how their 'energetics' would alter, or balance, the movement of *qi* in the body.

Herbalism in China — as in other herbal medicine traditions — can include non-plant material such as horn, hair, bone or skin of animals, reptiles, fish or birds. In general, the herbs would be infused, or decocted in the whole form, according to formulae, some of which have been in use for many centuries. Some ingredients are burned before adding the resultant ash to the formula. There is a growing herbal pharmaceutical industry in China, responding to the needs of exporters who are finding an increasing demand for the pills, tablets, syrups and decoctions that are still made from natural substances.

HERBAL MEDICINE IN THE AMERICAS

Slowly emerging into western consciousness is the herbal tradition of the native peoples of the Americas. This, too, is a tradition going back many centuries, possibly millennia. Written records, where they existed, were mostly destroyed by the invading Europeans four or five centuries ago, or they lie inaccessible in the Vatican archives, where most of the material that survived seems to have been deposited.

The language of a society displays basic elements of a culture's philosophy. While European languages are object-based, native American languages are process-based. Western societies are more concerned, philosophically, with definable, quantifiable material things. The native peoples of America speak of the ways to achieve a situation and the processes life entails. To this extent they, like the Chinese, are more focused on energy than on objects, on synthesis rather than analysis.

The four rites that are required for a medicine person to become fully initiated illustrate this difference. They are occasions, sometimes taking many weeks, when what is under 'examination' is not the person's temporary ability to remember facts, but that individual's ability to work with situations, to use intuition as well as knowledge, to access the spirit. To this extent, the word 'medicine' has a quite different meaning for a native American than it does for a European. It is a word that shows up the inadequacy of one linguistic form to translate accurately into another. To a native American, *medicine* seems to describe the effect caused by an event, an encounter, or an interaction of people, or animals, or plants, or any combination of these, or other creatures. The interaction of the spirits of all creatures is equally important to them.

Unique to the Aboriginal peoples of all continents, especially the Americas and Australia, is the sense they have that all life and all phenomena are an integral part of one another and should be respected as such. Their intention of love, respect and gratitude towards all and for all other life forms is not found widely in the west. Westerners find this attitude of respect — it is so hard to find a word that truly expresses the intention — alien, rather than alienating. However, some modern western practitioners are beginning to use prayers, meditations and visualisations that bring the same intention to bear on what they've taken from the plant or animal world and what they are mediating for their clients.

EUROPEAN HERBALISM

European herbalism has a different history from the Chinese or the Aboriginal. From a state of integration with cosmic phenomena, when each herb — each creature — had a known affinity to a planet, the knowledge and practice of herbalism became an outlawed, suspect aspect of the occult, only to rise again during the twentieth century. To Galen, or Paracelsus, or more recently Gerard or Culpeper, the plants of field and wayside had many and varied uses as foods, as remedies and as household commodities. The many that have fallen into disuse are unfortunately assumed by most of the population to be poisonous.

The traditions of herbal healing in China and India and among the indigenous peoples of America were not confined to women, unlike in Europe. There were other differences too, because the non-European traditions were concerned with the balancing of energies, rather than the simple physical adjustment on which the European culture seems to have concentrated. In the Americas, in China and in India, healing techniques — including the use of herbs — were augmented by the use of meditation, prayer and ritual. Thus the notion of context is extended beyond the physical world into the esoteric. And why not? We all know how different our moods can be under different weather conditions. If we can be affected by something so apparently ephemeral as the weather, why shouldn't plant medication be enhanced by blessed intention?

It is only among the indigenous cultures — like the women and their work, suppressed and outlawed for hundreds of years — that esotericism allied to healing has survived and is now re-surfacing to augment the relationship we can have with our natural, physical context.

ORTHODOX MEDICINE AND MEDIEVAL HERBALISM

Modern orthodox medicine grew, to some extent, out of medieval herbalism. The plant derivatives *digitalis* — from foxgloves — and *belladonna* — from deadly nightshade — are still used, although they are now chemically reproduced in the laboratory, rather than harvested in the field. Both can kill if used without an understanding of their strength. *Digitalis* slows the heartbeat and *belladonna* induces sleep that can lead to coma and death. There are very few plants — weeds or otherwise — that have poisonous qualities, but because there are some, it is wise to be guided by good books on plant identification, for want of a human expert. If in doubt, don't use! But for every potentially poisonous plant, there are hundreds of plants that are not only safe, but actively beneficial.

THE INDUSTRIALISATION OF WESTERN MEDICINE

The analytical European mind sought ever more finite detail, until 'active ingredients' were eventually isolated from their plant sources. The end result was that the original sources became — and remain — unrecognisable. Penicillin, the first antibiotic, was developed from a mould that grows on bread. The first contraceptive pill was developed from a plant used for centuries by Paraguayan women to prevent child-bearing. Morphine, a potent pain-killer, was originally derived from the opium poppy. Analytical science has reached the stage where it can forego the use of the original plant and instead create the active ingredients in the laboratory from chemicals. What it has so far failed to do is to re-create the spirit of the original plant, or to see any necessity to do so.

The development of orthodox physical medicine in the west has moved away from the cosmic integration of previous centuries into the use of many substances that are designed to kill. 'Anti-biotic' means 'anti-life-thing', for example. In addition, the fact that chemotherapy and radiotherapy (or radiation treatment) can and sometimes does kill the cancer's host is usually overlooked.

Doctors are no longer trained to make up a medicine for a patient. They are instead dependent on a highly competitive, organised range of multi-national businesses, whose prime motivation is profit. Using animals that in no way resemble humans, they impart and create painful diseases in order to see if some substance they are developing can 'cure', or not. The two polarities of medical outlook could not be further apart, the one accenting the equal integrity of all living things, the other the domination of all things by humans for material prizes.

However, medical science is finding that isolating the active ingredient and using it over a period of time can have unexpected and often unwelcome results. For example, strains of bacteria have evolved that are impervious to penicillin; the derivative from the Paraguayan contraceptive plant caused thrombosis in many women, whereas it had never done so used in its natural state. Yet the authoritarian stance of orthodox medicine is such that many people believe there is no alternative to having what is prescribed by their GP, or the specialist to whom they are sent.

THE GROWTH OF THE DOMINATOR CULTURE

While the industrialisation of medicine was taking place, herbalism was becoming relegated to folklore. It came to be considered the purview of country women, who by definition were unsophisticated, uneducated, unreliable and suspected of occult practices. These truly *wise* women were once the health carers for each community in Europe. The growth of the dominator culture, and in particular the dominator Church, began the denigration that turned into physical abuse of the wise women, who were perceived as witches, creatures of evil fit only to be killed. During the religious Inquisition in Europe, and at the beginning of the Age of Reason, thousands of women were killed, for no better reason than their use of natural substances to treat illness and disease — as well as their observation of the spirit. While thousands of women died, the dominating religion and the growing schools of (male) doctors and scientists increased their power over society during the seventeenth and eighteenth centuries.

Though much died out with the murdered women, some knowledge survived, passed secretly from mother to daughter, so that in the latter part of the twentieth century the knowledge and the empowerment that goes with it are surfacing again in a more intellectually liberal climate. Herbalism's gentle nurturance is returning, if not to the mainstream of medicine, at least as a strand in the many-textured fabric of the intuitive, wholistic health practices that are challenging the grip of industrialised, chemical therapies.

Although men took over and calibrated and compartmentalised the nurturing, healing skills of women, some relics of the ancient concept of context and inclusiveness of all phenomena remained. In many of the older 'herbals' by Galen, Gerard, or Culpeper, herbs are designated under one or another Zodiacal sign. Advice is also given on harvesting individual herbs under specific phases of the moon. These wholly valid conditions, which have largely been dismissed by the more recent scientific fraternity, can be borne out by most gardeners, who know that plants thrive better under a waxing moon — because the energy is increasing — and less as she wanes. Similarly, plants are better harvested in dry conditions in the earlier half of the day, before noon — again, when the energy is increasing.

A MODERN HERBAL

While the renowned herbalists of the past have all been men, there is a notable herbal book compiled by a woman. In the 1930s, Mrs M. Grieve's book, *A Modern Herbal* was first published. In it she included the most comprehensive body of work about almost every known medicinal herb in both Europe and North America. Mrs Grieve gave botanical details (though not comprehensive illustrations), many colloquial names, historical background, medicinal uses, parts of the plants used and in what form as well as scientific analyses of the chemical constituents. A truly monumental work, the book has never been out of print since its first publication.

HERBAL MEDICINE AND HOMEOPATHY

Rooted in herbalism is one of the other wholistic disciplines: homeopathy. Whereas eastern medicine uses mostly water-based processes for utilising the virtues of plant parts, the European tradition also uses an alcohol-based extractive process — the tincture. This process releases not only the allopathic energy of the plant — the cure by opposites — to some degree, but also the homeopathic virtue of like cures like. No tincture works as a homeopathic potency would, as that requires a rhythmic agitation (known as succession), as well as dilution, but the basic potential is present.

CONCLUSION

Analytical science has defined most of the substances that compose each plant and has thus refined our ability to understand the potential of the plants at our disposal. A brilliant chef doesn't need to know the detailed vitamin and trace-element content of the foods he or she cooks; by the same token, lay herbalists — who may also be superb cooks! — are able to use plants to enhance health and to adjust ill-health, just as our ancestors did, using empirical knowledge and experience.

CHAPTER THREE

Why Alternatives are Needed

ALLERGIC REACTIONS

When I was a girl and I was given penicillin, I was described in the doctor-speak of the time as 'having a reaction' to it. Today, an allergy to penicillin is referred to as such and if you are ever hospitalised you are asked whether you have it or not. The sensitive area today is steroids. Yet in this case, the onus is removed from the individual and placed on the medication: it has 'side-effects'.

If you have an allergy to penicillin, when a doctor wishes to treat you for a condition that appears to her or him to require an antibiotic, you will be offered an antibiotic other than penicillin. If you are allergic to one antibiotic, however, it may be that you will also be allergic to others, even if they are not genetically related to the original one. You should also bear in mind that your children are likely to inherit your allergies and your tendencies. This usually follows the Mendel theory — that sons inherit from their mothers and daughters from their fathers.

Today, the allergy I have to penicillin has another classification. It is called anaphylaxis. This term has come into prominence, not through the allergies manifested to medications alone, but more commonly to allergic reactions to food stuffs. The most widely known is an allergy to peanuts. Also implicated are all other nuts, fish, milk and milk products, eggs and wasp and bee stings. Sometimes an individual has eaten the substance many times before without having any allergic reaction. Equally, they may have taken penicillin, or received wasp or bee stings without previously having an allergic reaction.

If an initial, fairly mild, reaction is ignored, the next time the body encounters the allergen, the reaction may be more dramatic. In some very sensitive people, the reaction can be very severe the first time. Mild, or severe, the allergic reaction to these substances is called *anaphylactic shock*. It can kill. People with such allergies should wear some prominent piece of jewellery, a pendant or a bangle, engraved with their problem. They should also contact the Anaphylaxis Campaign, listed in 'Helpful Addresses', page 117.

HERBAL ALTERNATIVES

Doctors find it very hard to come up with alternatives to antibiotics and it is often up to the individual who experiences an allergy to find an alternative treatment. Effective internal cleansers to use as replacements are: Garlic, Burdock, Sheep Sorrel, Comb Honey or Lemon, Fennel, Cinnamon, Sage, Rosemary and others. External cleansers include Hydrogen Peroxide — super-oxygenated water — Comb Honey, Periwinkle, St John's Wort and Tea-tree (oil). If an external wound or infection is the problem, always use an internal cleanser as well as an external one.

THE EFFECT OF CHEMICALS ON FOOD AND ON PEOPLE

Although I have seen no scientific report to bear out the theory, it seems to me that while the human body has taken generations to adapt to different food stuffs in their natural, organic state, it has not had the time to adapt to exposure of foods to toxic chemicals. The toxic chemicals to which I refer are the chemicals used in farming. They are intended to be toxic only to the insects, 'weeds' or fungi against which they are used. Chemical fertilisers are intended to make the crop grow faster and larger.

In addition, chemical fertilisers are now developed in tandem with hybridised seeds, so that any one hybrid will only respond to one particular chemical fertiliser — a wonder of modern science, until you realise that the hybrid seed, like the hybrid animal commonly known as a 'mule' — is incapable of breeding. The use of such seed means therefore that no fertile seed can be reserved from any year's crop — it has to be bought, every year. This is resulting in the banning of fertile, reserved seed by governments who have signed the GATT (Global Agreement on Tariffs and Trade) Treaty, while the hybrid-fertiliser tandem is put in its place. I hereby re-designate the initial letters to mean Global Attack on Traditional Trading. Hybridised seed, whatever form of fertiliser it responds to, because it is unable to reproduce itself after the first generation, lacks life force; therefore it is ultimately less nourishing than its fertile ancestors, from which it has been bred.

I believe that the human body has found it very difficult to adapt to all these chemicals. If it takes minute quantities of hormonal chemicals to have profound effects on the body, how much more profound are the effects of these non-human derived chemicals, in grosser amounts, likely to be? That the body reacts adversely to these chemicals is widely accepted; that the body cannot differentiate the chemical allergen from the food vehicle with which it originally identified does not seem to have been considered. 'Let your food be your medicine ...'

CHAPTER FOUR

Harvesting

WHAT TO PICK

With your chosen plant identification book in hand (first law of botanists: take the book to the plant, not the plant to the book), go to the area where you expect to find the plant(s) you want to harvest. If you want to use fresh plant material for any particular condition, first check that the condition has arisen at the optimum time of the year for harvesting the plant material you seek!

If you are searching for flowers or leaves, pick only the best specimens and never pick all you find, especially if the plant is an annual, like Eyebright. Unless there are plants left to seed, you will have no crop to search for next year. If roots are your harvest, dig up the best looking plants. As a general rule, roots are best dug in autumn, after the plant has flowered and fruited and the leaves are beginning to die back. Apart from roots, it is usually possible to pick a few flowers, or leaves, or fruit and leave the plant relatively unimpaired. This is the ideal. However, if your chosen harvest is Burdock, for example, make sure you dig up only the plants that haven't developed the prickly seed carriers that give the plant its name. With Burdock, a biennial plant, it is only the root of the first year's growth that is used.

Check these sorts of details, and remember to pick only what you need.

You also need to bear in mind that in some countries there are laws to protect plants that grow in the wild. In the United Kingdom, it is illegal to pick any part of any wild plant. In Ireland, only some plants are protected by

law. On the other hand, house-builders and road-makers
have no such proscription placed on their activities. So, if
you discover earth-movers about to move on to a bit of
land that is host to any plants, however rare, dig them up
and transplant them to a safe, but similar environment in
the hope that they will grow on. Failing this, harvest all
you can find, with impunity.

If you have a garden, or even a window box, you may
wish to grow medicinal herbs for yourself. Seeds of wild
plants, often organically propagated, are available from
specialist suppliers, some of whom are listed in 'Helpful
Addresses', pages 117–18.

If you are already a gardener, beginning to branch into
medicinal self-help, look carefully at every plant before
you weed it out of your cultivated beds. You may find
useful plants, such as Spear-Leaf Plantain, or Lamb's
Tongue Sorrel, or some other useful culinary or medicinal
plant that has honoured you by choosing to grow there.
Most of these plants will transplant well. On the other
hand, you may like to let them remain where they have
chosen to grow.

WHERE TO PICK

This is a concern that seriously reduces the number of
sites where harvests can be made. It is really easier to state
where not to pick.

Avoid roadside verges and hedgerows, because of the
damaging fall-out from vehicle exhausts, lead, sulphur, etc.
In addition, avoid anywhere within 110 yards (100
metres) of high-tension electric wires, or within the same
distance of any form of radio or radar transmitter, or
within sight — no matter how far distant — of any
microwave transmitter. Within ten miles of any nuclear

power station all plant life will be impaired in some way, or will have absorbed something harmful by its proximity to the polluting agent. The same applies to any plant within five miles of an industrial production unit with a chimney.

Similarly, it is inadvisable to harvest plant life from land that has been subjected to any form of chemical fertiliser or weed-, insect- or fungus-killer, or the banks or hedgerows surrounding any fields so treated. Even if the plants have survived the onslaught, many of them will have absorbed some part of the substances; these may prove poisonous to people, or in some cases cause an allergic reaction — quite the opposite from what you might intend!

You will get to know the area in which you live very well and you may have to travel quite a distance to find plants in optimum health. Of course, this only means the best you can find. *No* plant is now as healthy as plants were before industrialised, chemical farming, the Chernobyl nuclear accident, atomic bomb testing, or the increase in ultraviolet light coming through the holes in the ozone layer. In so far as the last is concerned, some plants are now what is called UV Indicators, because their germination rate has been adversely affected by the increase in ultraviolet light in such a way as to make the degree of irradiation quantifiable. In a similar way, the incidence of different forms of lichen can be used to determine not only the degree of industrial pollution, but the type of chemical in each case.

So, the advice is, provided all the criteria already listed are observed, pick away on any land where you have permission. Don't omit to ask, because not only is it discourteous, but in many parts of the British Isles it is also an illegal trespass.

WHEN TO PICK

This is easy! To obtain flowers, leaves and fruit for drying, or otherwise processing into medicaments, pick only in fine weather, when the plant material has no dew or rain drops on it and before noon. Make sure the flowers and the fruit are in peak condition, open to their fullest extent — or just about to be — at their ripest and with unbroken skin. Leaves should be picked just as the buds of the annual flowering are beginning to show. After this, the energies of the plant will go into the flowers in preparation for fruiting and the moment will have been lost. This is particularly relevant to the smaller annual and perennial herbs, such as the Mint family, Sage, etc.

Evergreen leaves, such as Periwinkle, can be picked as needed. Seeds such as Nasturtium should be gathered before the frosts begin and the succulent tendrils of the plant die off. However, the fruit of the bushes, Wild Rose, the Hip and White Thorn and Black Thorn (Haw and Sloe respectively) should all be left to harvest *after* the first frosts, because the fibres of the fruit are softened and the sugar content is improved by the frost.

Occasionally, bark is gathered — from the Slippery Elm, for instance. In this case, it's the bark of the twigs that is gathered in late spring-time, before the leaf has begun to form. If the bark of the trunk or the major branches is taken, especially if it is taken from all around the trunk or branch, then the tree will die.

HOW TO PICK

For flowers such as Roses, Dandelion heads, Primroses, Violets, Celandines and so on, use gentle fingers. For the umbilliferae — flowers that grow in clusters of tiny florets, such as Elder or Meadowsweet — use scissors and cut the stalk 4–6 inches behind the flowering head. Do not handle these delicate flowering heads, because they bruise very easily while they are fresh, which can ruin them for use.

In bundles of half-a-dozen or so, place the heads inside a large, wide-open brown paper bag and seal the mouth of the bag around the stalks with a loop of string, or cord. Such bags are readily available from any paper wholesaler, or perhaps you can persuade a friendly retailer to get 1,000 for you of the largest size available. They are not expensive and can be used over and over again if you are careful, so they are a good investment.

Carry your harvest home with the loops suspended from your fingers to avoid crushing the flowers, although they are less likely to be bruised once they are protected by the paper. Hang the bags in a warm atmosphere away from direct heat or direct light. If you have a clothes airer, especially the old fashioned sort that hangs from the ceiling, this is an ideal place for the flowers to dry.

Another idea is to suspend the bags along the bars of clothes hangers and then hook the hangers over the top of the airing-cupboard door, leaving that door ajar. An attic or spare bedroom is equally good, provided the atmosphere is dry and warm and there is some sort of ventilation. Flowers thus treated will dry within a week; some leaves, which can be treated in the same way, may need a little longer. Colt's Foot, for example, I find takes about ten days to become crisp.

Ideally, harvest all you can by hand. If there is any risk of uprooting a plant by using that technique, then use scissors or a really sharp knife. A box or a flat-bottomed basket is useful to carry the harvest home from the site in order to prevent crushing. The golden rule is *never* to use plastic bags, because plant material sweats while it's fresh

and this will cause decomposition to begin very rapidly.
The moisture that will gather on the plant will also defeat
the object of picking when the plant is completely dry.

DRYING THE HARVEST

I have already mentioned umbilliferae. Handle any harvest
as little as possible, and get it either into bags that are hung
straight away, or spread onto clean sheets on a flat surface
such as a bed, or the floor of a room that isn't used. You
can make very simple drying cabinets, based on the
vegetable dehydrators so common in rural America.

If the drying takes place with the minimum of
movement of the harvest and not in direct light, then the
colour will be retained in the plants. To maintain this, it is
important to store your dried harvest in air-tight
containers, when the harvest is completely dry. If the walls
of the container are transparent, then line the jars with
brown paper.

Roots need to be washed carefully after harvesting. Pat
them dry before chopping them small and spreading them
thinly on a flat baking sheet. Roots are the only harvest
that can be put in the oven which should be at a low
temperature. If you are drying Dandelion root for a coffee
substitute, however, then a hot oven is ideal because
charring enhances the flavour!

Always label with the name of the plant and the date
of harvest. Keep the containers out of the reach of
children, away from direct light and heat but in a dry
place. You may then use your harvest as and when you
wish.

CHAPTER FIVE

What Conditions Can You Treat?

Depending on how far you have jumped over the confidence barrier, you may decide to treat a variety of ailments or conditions yourself. A number of conditions are better given self-treatment in any case.

WHAT CONDITIONS RESPOND TO HERBAL MEDICATION?

Childhood diseases such as: chicken pox, German measles, measles, mumps, scarlet fever or whooping cough; the common cold, a chill, or a feverish cold (usually, incorrectly, referred to as flu); simple digestive disorders of elimination, diarrhoea or constipation; septic wounds or ulcers: all will respond to herbal treatment. These are simple, though often painful and distressing, disorders and diseases. They are dealt with under the section on disorders and what to treat them with.

It is *not enough*, however, to use herbal, or any other form of treatment, without appropriate nursing. Nursing doesn't only mean bed care, but the correct way to clean and dress wounds and how to feed and water infected folk.

One of the conditions that responds well to herbal treatment is Candidiasis, as outlined in detail below.

CANDIDIASIS

THE IMMUNE SYSTEM

AIDS (Acquired Immune Deficiency Syndrome) first focused the modern human mind on the immune system.

This complex entity is a mutual dependency of a healthy blood supply, supported by elastic and absorbent lungs and by a digestive system that has a proper balance of bacteria and fungi living within it — 4–6 lbs of bacteria and fungi, in fact. This is a weight equal to that of a vital organ. These creatures lead a symbiotic existence in our guts and play a considerable role in the healthy process of digestion and elimination. If these three bodily systems — the blood supply, the lungs and the digestive system — are all functioning normally, then the actual front-line agents of immunity, the T-cells in the blood, perform their job and we remain healthy. As soon as any one of the three basic systems becomes impaired, the T-cells start to falter and no longer provide the protection from disease that nature intends.

What is Candidiasis?

Candidiasis is a condition for which there is no known clinical test, which has meant that it has taken longer than it might have for this phenomenon to be recognised. Its manifestation is directly linked to damage inflicted on the large colony of fungi and bacteria that exists in the gut. This damage has been found to be caused by both direct and indirect medication; the medicines in question cover two ranges — antibiotics and steroids. Direct medication is what your doctor prescribes for you. It has been established that one single course of antibiotics in any twelve-month period is the maximum 'safe' dose for the average person. Remember that few of us are average! Your body may tolerate more, or it may tolerate less.

The Endocrine System

Steroids is the name given to hormones that are administered as medication. Hormones are the name for a vast complex of highly sophisticated chemicals that the body produces naturally and in minute quantities. The endocrine system, which produces these substances, has a built-in set of fail-safe triggers that have to respond before an activating hormone is released. The master-gland that appears to orchestrate most of the fail-safe triggers is the pituitary gland, in harmony with the hypothalamus. This tiny gland — the size of a pea in an adult — controls five other glands: the ovary/testis, the mammary, the adrenal and the thyroid, as well as bones, skin and the kidneys. Of these, let's look at the adrenal as an example. The two sections of this pair of glands (one is situated over each of the two kidneys), the medulla and the cortex, between them control the brain, the pupils of the eye, muscles, lungs, heart, stomach, intestines and the metabolic absorption and release of carbohydrates and fatty acids.

The endocrine system has seven sites in the body, which can be described as the 'chemical' centres. Each is closely associated with a nerve plexus, which in turn can be called an 'electrical' centre. (Each of these pairs of endocrine/nerve plexus couples is exactly positioned to relate to one of the seven chakras, the 'wheels' or vortices of energy that link the physical body, through its electro-magnetic field — also known as the aura — to the cosmic energy that links all living beings. The chakra system is an important part of Indian and Chinese religious and medical practice.)

Steroids are manufactured in the laboratory from chemical 'look-alikes' that resemble the natural chemicals produced in the body by the endocrine system. No administration of steroids can ever be as precise as the self-administration of hormones by a healthy body.

The effect of direct medication of antibiotics and

steroids, which includes all varieties of contraceptive pill, is to upset the balance of fungi, bacteria and hormonal secretions. If this balance is severely upset by, say, repeated courses of antibiotics, or long-term use of contraceptive pills, steroid inhalers, or hydro-cortisone creams, for example, then Candidiasis is one of the most common outcomes.

INDIRECT MEDICATION

Indirect medication is used to describe human absorption of medication that has been administered to other creatures, that humans have absorbed by eating those creatures. Steroids and antibiotics fed to cattle, sheep, poultry and farmed fish can be the cause of Candidiasis in people who have never previously had reason to visit their doctor and for whom that doctor has never prescribed either antibiotic or steroid preparations.

The incidence of minor to severe Candidiasis in western populations is widespread and the classic example of how herbal care can act both as prophylactic (preventative) and healer. If, in all food selection, organic and locally grown/caught vegetables, meats and fish are chosen, indirect medication is immediately ruled out. Organic food is expensive and can be hard to find, but the more people demand it the more will be produced and the cheaper and more accessible it will become.

If we learn about our bodies, and especially learn how to listen to our bodily reactions, we can come to know when it is necessary to use material (herbal) healing substances; when it is necessary to use techniques that balance the energy systems such as homeopathy, acupuncture, or acupressure; when we need someone to listen to us during counselling or a workshop environment that can release what we feel is blocked.

Symptoms of Candidiasis

The possible symptoms are listed on the left, and herbal methods of treating them are on the right:

MENTAL AND EMOTIONAL SYMPTOMS	TREATMENTS
Depression and lack of self-worth Loss of short-term memory Inability to concentrate Indecisiveness	Mental and emotional symptoms adjust to treatment by energy-balancing techniques, in conjunction with herbal treatment of the physical symptoms. Sometimes they are self adjusting when herbal and dietary treatments alone are used.

PHYSICAL SYMPTOMS	
Recurrently sore throat	2 drops of Sandalwood oil in half a glass of warm water, gargled.
Recurrently itchy eyes	2 drops of Rescue Remedy or Five Flower Essence in a quarter glass of warm water, used as an eye-bath or an infusion of Eyebright as an eye-bath (see Recipe section for making an infusion).
Recurrently itchy ears	As for itchy eyes, wash out the ears.
Unexplained rashes	If these are itchy, Five Flower

Cream, or Rescue Cream, applied as frequently as necessary; or an infusion of Goosegrass, also known as Cleavers.

Recurrent fungal infections (the most common is Thrush, which can occur in the mouth, around the genitals, in the armpits and around the finger and toenails, but not usually all at once!)

Aloe Gel, straight out of the leaf from your Aloe Vera plant; or a wash or douche using infused Marigold, or Garlic, *or* Ground Ivy; *or* a wash or douche using 2 drops of Essential Oil of Thyme, Cinnamon or Savory, or Tea-tree in warm water; *or* (applied undiluted) Gentian Violet 1% (an Aniline Dye, not a herbal preparation).

Recurrent cystitis

Stop eating all acidic foods, including all citrus fruits (except lemon), potatoes, peppers, chillies and tomatoes and stop drinking tea and coffee, except one weak cup per day to prevent withdrawal symptoms. Drink copious amounts of an infusion of Linseed; remember to strain it, unless you are also constipated. Drink and douche with an infusion of any one of the following: Butterbur, Celery, Chickweed, Comfrey, Elderflower, Goosegrass, Horsetail, Lady's Mantle, Meadowsweet, Nettle, Red Clover; or douche with 2 drops of any of the following essential oils, in warm

	water: Juniper, Parsley Seed, Sandalwood.
Constipation	Drink lots of warm or cool water and infusions of Bogbean, or Chickweed, or Comfrey. Eat rhubarb, stewed apples or pears and squat on the lavatory, concentrating on the need to eliminate, *without straining*. Squatting is better than sitting — if you can't get your feet onto the lavatory seat, buy a bowl and squat over that, disposing of the contents down the lavatory when you've something to dispose of!
Diarrhoea	Drink a cup of hot milk with a level teaspoon of ground Cinnamon in it; or drink an infusion made from any one of the following: Bilberry, Blackberry, Comfrey, Meadowsweet, Raspberry, Tormentil, Yarrow; or drink warm water with two drops of either Cinnamon or Sage Essential Oil.

Diarrhoea and constipation may alternate.

TREATMENT WITH DIET

Candidiasis gets its name from one of the fungi in the gut, Candida albicans. Under healthy circumstances, this creature is held in check by the balanced population of other fungi and bacteria. Once this balance is disturbed, it can behave like dry-rot behaves in a house. Dry-rot starts as wet rot, say on a timber on which the spore has landed that is under a broken slate so that the rain comes in. The spore finds lots of damp to dissolve the food it needs contained in the wood and a nice warm environment because the timber gets warm in the area under the sun-heated slates.

One day someone repairs the broken slate, thus preventing the rain from entering anymore. Slowly the wood dries out, but the spore has grown to be quite a colony of mould which has eaten much of the wood sugars. When the wood is sufficiently dry, the panic which has taken hold of the now starving mould causes tendrils, called mycelia, to begin to grow out of the wood in an effort to find more wood to feed on. These mycelia can grow very long and they can penetrate stone and brick in their efforts to discover more wood. In extreme circumstances, this is what Candida albicans can do too. It can penetrate the walls of the gut in an effort to find a new environment. I would like to emphasise that this penetration happens only in very advanced and rare instances.

The diet is designed to starve the Candida albicans of the food that will cause it to continue its ravages and the foods that are excluded all contain either sugar or yeast, which is a fungus. This is a hard one, because this exclusion diet has to be maintained for at least six months and sometimes much longer.

You should eat: lots of leafy green vegetables, some cooked, some raw; plenty of grains: oats, barley, wheat, rice and pulses such as lentils, chick peas, beans and so on. Modest amounts of meat and fish can be eaten, but they must be from organic or natural sources. In other words, if it is impossible for your supplier to guarantee that the animals you want to eat the flesh of have not been given antibiotics or steroids in any form (these two substances are fed as a matter of course via prepared feeds for prophylactic reasons), you must not eat this flesh. Wild caught fish is safe, but farmed fish is not.

Eat lots of acidopholis-rich, unpasteurised natural yoghurt, which helps to replace some of the missing creatures that help to keep Candida albicans in check.

Sugar-bearing foods to leave out of your diet include:

- all fresh fruit
- all dried fruit
- all biscuits
- sugar
- jams
- all cakes
- all desserts
- all sweets.

Yeast-bearing foods to leave out of your diet include:

- all cheeses
- all yeast breads
- alcoholic drinks
- smoked fish
- smoked meats
- dried sausage, e.g. salami
- dried fruit
- vinegar
- mayonnaise
- soft fruit including grapes, strawberries, raspberries, bilberries, blackberries, plums, cherries and gooseberries
- yeast extracts (e.g. marmite).

Some Candidiasis sufferers find they can tolerate some yeast but no sugar-bearing foods without the symptoms flaring again, while some find the opposite. All Candidiasis sufferers should eat soda-bread, or unleavened bread. As time goes by — months in most instances — fruit can be re-introduced. It is wise to start with apples or pears, but *peel* them to be on the safe side and only eat them two or three times a week. Very gradually, other foods can also be re-introduced, like cottage cheese, but use discretion, don't pig out on Stilton, for example, or any other mould-rich — that is, fungus-rich — cheese.

It is probable that you will need to watch your diet for a long time. But the positive thing is that you may have found a wealth of good, safe things to eat that you never met before: 'Let your food be your medicine and your medicine be your food.'

CHAPTER SIX

Other Conditions to Treat

A charitable trust is being established with the intention of funding the creation of a peaceful, secluded place to which people who have received a diagnosis of terminal illness may go to escape the pressures of the medical orthodoxy, their well-meaning families and their friends, while they decide for themselves what form of treatment they would like and how they would choose to die. This is not about euthanasia — it is about the right to die with dignity, unencumbered by medical technology, or de-sensitised by orthodox medication.

Despite the western materialist fantasy that it is *not*, life is a terminal condition. I may never have a day's illness in my life, but, sometime, I will die. So will you. The trust is being created out of compassion. It would serve us well as individuals too if we considered our own attitude toward the treatment we would like to have and the sort of death we would choose, if we were ever to receive the sort of diagnosis that candidates for this retreat centre will face.

CANCER

The disease that is the most greatly feared and which a proportion as high as one quarter in the populations of technologically developed countries is subject to, is Cancer. While it is no longer surrounded by the secrecy that prevailed a generation ago — AIDS has taken its place in that regard — its diagnosis creates fear and panic on the part of the patient and distress and discomfort on the part of the medical practitioners who have to tell their patients

the news. In this climate of emotional cramp, people who
have had this diagnosis are often pushed into accepting
treatment they later wish they hadn't had. Some complain
of being refused the opportunity to make arrangements for
dependents in their families, or for substitutes in their
place of work, usually on the grounds that there's no time
like the present to get started on the treatment.

This is not to say the pressure from the medical
professionals is not being given with the best of intentions
and that they are fully conversant with the therapies they
use. Doctors are very highly trained and extremely
knowledgeable, but usually only in their specific
specialisation. Few of them expect anything but
compliance from their patients. Patients, on the other
hand, are often intimidated, not only by the shock of this
crisis, but also by the authoritarianism of their doctors.

A growing number of patients are having the courage
to say 'stop' and to refuse either the radiation therapy, or
the chemotherapy — the usual options offered. A nun said
to me recently, 'I think, if I had accepted the
chemotherapy I was offered, I would be dead by now.'
Another woman told me how enraged she was when she
discovered the burns and the pain and the loss of energy
that she experienced after having radiation treatment,
having been assured before the treatment began that there
would be no side-effects.

In addition, there is the pressure from and emotional
anxiety of friends and family, full of pain and anguish, all
with the best of intentions for the person diagnosed as
having Cancer.

A loved one has had the feared diagnosis. The
prognosis is poor. They stop and think about their
problem, examine all the options and decide to have

chemotherapy. Support them. Never undermine their decision once it is final, but supply them with all the information you can about the range of treatments that you can discover while they are still in the decision making process. You may find some of the books in 'Recommended Reading' helpful at this time.

RESEARCH INTO CANCER

In 1963, a thirty-five-year-old biologist called Jerard Hurwitz, living and working in the United States, was awarded a Cancer research grant of $692,000 to provide him with funds for his experiments and to pay the salaries of his assistants and himself for thirty-four years. This was announced in a brief article in the *New York World Telegram and Sun* of Saturday 14 December of that year; the last two paragraphs of the article make chilling reading:

> There is one catch clause in the grant. Should a cure for Cancer be discovered during the next thirty-four years, the grant will be terminated.

On this point, Dr Hurwitz jokes:

> Some people must think that all the people looking into the disease have signed a blood pact not to announce a cure until they are all on their death beds so the grants will continue.

Dr Hurwitz is only one among many thousands of people involved in Cancer research before and since that award was made. There is an enormous amount of money spent on — and earned — by research and manufacture of drugs used in the treatment of Cancer. The pharmaceutical companies that do this work are large, mostly what are called multinational, having manufacturing units in more than one country. Most pharmaceutical companies also manufacture agricultural chemicals — they are businesses that intend, and succeed, in making huge profits for their shareholders.

TREATMENT FOR CANCER

While the pharmaceutical companies, charities and business investors are funding researchers like Dr Hurwitz, there are other people working independently to find answers to the problems of Cancer. Some of them have established clinics in which they use the preparations they have developed to treat those with Cancer. Many of these treatments involve concerns about an appropriate diet, vitamin and mineral supplements to that diet — and herbal remedies.

Thousands of people who have received orthodox chemotherapy and radiation therapy have recovered from their Cancer. We all know, however, of others who have died, sometimes from the effects of these very therapies. Yet we tend to assume they died of Cancer, because that was what they, and we, had been told they were going to die from.

There are also thousands of people who have benefited from herbal and unorthodox treatments who have recovered from Cancer. Some have died, but of these, many have found an unorthodox therapy that has allowed them to die with dignity and, often, free from pain. We hear far less about these forms of treatment. Some of them are very simple and inexpensive and can be prepared in any family kitchen. There are also people who have tried to exploit others' fear and who have charged large sums for some of these remedies. This is hardly surprising, as we have plenty of role-models for greed.

THE DIFFERENCE BETWEEN ORTHODOX AND UNORTHODOX TREATMENTS

The fundamental difference between orthodox and any alternative treatment for Cancer is the same philosophical one that exists between these treatments for any other disorder. Because of the magnitude of Cancer, though, it is much starker.

Orthodox treatment stems from the analytical research, quantifiable testing techniques and confidence in technology that permeates the whole of western culture. It focuses on the disorder and loses sight of the individual experiencing that disorder. On the other hand, the unorthodox or alternative adopts primarily a wholistic approach. Therefore attention will be paid not only to the size and frequency of doses of medication, but also to dietary and environmental factors, as well as to the choices of the person with the problem.

Using liberally the language of warfare, orthodox treatment of Cancer is actually designed to 'kill' the 'invading' cancer cells. Like all military operations, a lot of 'innocent' cells will be killed at the same time, sometimes resulting in the 'victory' of the 'battle' but the loss of the 'war'.

Unorthodox treatment of Cancer comes from a different philosophy, where harmony and the enhancement of the individual's well-being and ability of the body to re-adopt its own protection from illness, are the prime motivating factors. There is a daily recognition of the individual's state of mind and body that will mean treatment will be selected — or not — according to their wishes. If they are going to die, no all-out effort will be made to cause painful delay. The hospice movement has done an enormous amount to begin to effect a change in the attitudes of orthodox doctors to this dilemma of the recognition of a need for dignified death.

If the decision is made to rely on unorthodox treatment, then you or your loved one have demolished the confidence barrier — but you will also need the full support of your family and friends. In the chapter with recipes for herbal medications, there is one which has proved highly successful in treating disorders that result from a severely damaged immune system and especially Cancer. It is called Essiac. Essiac is not a cure for Cancer, but many people who have taken it when they have had Cancer have had great benefit from it.

In addition, there is a herb that can be infused to make a 'tea' which marvellously relieves pain. It is called hemp. Illegal, it is better known by its Latin name, Cannabis sativa. There is a movement to legalise it for medicinal use.

CHAPTER SEVEN

How to Give Treatment

PREREQUISITES FOR TREATMENT

Most treatment of diseases, disorders and accidents amounts to common sense. Unfortunately, we have become slovenly in our use of this sense and it is now quite *un*common. Maybe because we have been conditioned to rely on experts and what we're told are miracle cures — by which I mean antibiotics and steroids — most people no longer think of the first practical requisite for *any* treatment: hygiene. Whatever you have just been doing, if you are answering the call of someone who is ill, coping with an accident, or just picking up the baby, *wash your hands first.*

The second most important essential is TLC — Tender Loving Care. This starts at the door of the room, or the moment you see the person you've arrived to help and it takes the form of a smile. Be warm and gentle. Inspire confidence by being thorough and methodical and, where appropriate, give big hugs and little kisses.

You have to remember that these two basic essentials need to be observed after your ministrations are over, as well. You leave the room, the scene of the accident, wherever, with a smile and words of confidence, and you *wash your hands.*

NURSING

Whatever form of treatment you are providing, the one practice that relates to many accidents, all infections and many recurrent or chronic conditions is nursing. Apart from the profession of nursing — largely used in hospitals — no one is taught how to nurse at home in a lay capacity. It's hard work, but it makes both the sufferer and the carer feel better.

If you intend to provide your own medical care using herbs and allied remedies, you are going to have to do it in the home. In the absence of fever, keep the sufferer warm. For nursing a fever, see below.

NATURAL FIBRES

People with a fever will perspire when the fever 'breaks', and their sheets and pillow covers will need to be changed frequently — maybe two or three times a day. Usually this stage doesn't last more than a day or two, unless some chronically febrile condition is involved. It is far more comfortable for the sufferer if you use pure cotton, or linen sheets, not nylon or polyester. Try to keep a couple of pairs as part of your emergency kit, especially if you have children. Scatter Lavender heads or Bog Myrtle leaves through them when you fold them to store. Or scatter a few drops of Lavender or Rosemary essential oil over them. This not only smells fragrant, it helps to keep insects away and induces rest for the sick person when the sheets come to be used.

Cotton or linen should also be the material used for the nightdresses or pyjamas that the sick person wears. The reason for this is that no man-made fibre has yet been invented that achieves the same as a natural fibre. Natural fibres ventilate the body. Secretions such as perspiration can pass through the fibre and evaporate. This doesn't happen with man-made fibre. Instead, the secretions settle in or on the fibre and the heat of the body sets up a bacteriological decomposition which rapidly gets smelly!

The bacteria can then transfer to infect the surrounding skin. Arctic explorers get very few opportunities to change their clothes, so leaders of Arctic expeditions forbid their team to wear man-made fibre clothing, because of the smelly factor.

It is helpful to remember that of the natural fibres, vegetable fibres — cotton and linen — tend to be cooling, while wool, silk, alpaca, mohair, camel and all other hairs are derived from animals that are warming. So feather/down duvets, or woollen blankets, are recommended for the sick bed, too.

NURSING A FEVER

If the sick person has a fever, or the weather is hot and there's a risk of them over-heating, keep them cool. It's much easier to keep warm than it is to keep cool. Wiping a perspiring person with a cool, damp sponge creates evaporation at the skin level and evaporation brings the temperature down. Take care not to allow the person to get chilled after sponging. Dry them carefully and clothe them in dry clothing.

During a fever, drink is more important than food. The skin is not just a wrapper to keep our insides in; it's the largest organ of elimination the body has and it loses enormous amounts of body fluids through perspiration. Dehydration when a fever is present is even more dangerous than when there is no fever, so the fluid balance must be maintained. The best drink at all stages of sickness and recovery is water — fresh spring water if possible — but if that is unobtainable, use uncarbonated, bottled spring water, served at room temperature, without ice. Little and often is far better than pints at long intervals, so a covered jug should be placed beside the bed with a glass — unless the sufferer is too young to cope alone.

There's a fine line between breaking the confidence barrier and being too sure of yourself. If the sufferer has a persistent high temperature, or simultaneous vomiting and diarrhoea and either has lasted for more than twenty-four hours, call a doctor. If the sick person is less than three years of age, wait no longer than twelve hours. Meanwhile, at the onset of either condition, but especially the vomiting and/or diarrhoea, give the following mixture instead of plain water. It is designed to remedy dehydration and to restore the body's natural acidity level.

To 7 pt/3 litres hot, boiled spring water, add the following (stir and dissolve well):

- 10 teaspoonfuls of honey or cane sugar
- ½ a teaspoonful of salt
- ½ a teaspoonful of bicarbonate of soda.

Cool this mixture, and give little and often — in teaspoonfuls if necessary. Do this whether you call the doctor or not. A good way to prevent many digestive disorders is to make it a family rule that everyone, adult or child, washes their hands in soap and water *every* time they use the toilet, even if it's only for a pee!

NURSING INFECTIOUS DISEASES

In infectious diseases like mumps, measles or chicken pox, any drink other than water feels like pure acid and makes the salivary glands in the mouth secrete most painfully. So in these cases water is definitely best. Milk may seem to be a bland alternative, but in fact it is not a good idea on two counts. Firstly, it forms mucous and can give the sufferer problems because of it. Secondly, almost all milk is pasteurised. This process involves heating the milk very fast before cooling it again, also very fast, in order to kill bacteria, especially tuberculosis. The problem is that the heating process also destroys *helpful* bacteria and enzymes that exist naturally in the milk and actively assist in the digestive process. Therefore, much of the life force of the milk has been eliminated before it ever reaches your table.

People with measles risk damage to their eyes even in ordinary daylight. For the duration of the fever stage and for the first few days following the outbreak of the rash, they *must not* watch television, or have the curtains of the room open, or the light on. They certainly mustn't be allowed to read.

DIET FOR THOSE CONFINED TO BED

Foods for people without a fever but confined to bed should include predominately repair foods, rich in proteins, vitamins, trace minerals and life force. Avoid foods that produce quick energy bursts, such as sugars, heavy pies or puddings and fried food. Use high protein foods, such as lamb's liver, or rice and chick peas, but in small amounts, or as soups. Use onion and garlic as much as possible, especially garlic. Scramble eggs, or serve omelette with small amounts of bread or toast.

Use lots of fresh, leafy vegetables, steamed and/or raw, although raw vegetables should be only in very small proportions to the rest of the menu and always finely chopped. A plate with a small amount of colourful, carefully prepared food is much more likely to be returned empty, possibly with a request for a second helping, than a plate with a large amount of sloppily prepared food. It is in caring for the sick that 'do as you would be done by' comes into its own! Fresh fruit is preferable to cooked puddings, but always wash fruit very carefully, rinsing, finally, in spring water if possible. Natural yoghurt, unsweetened, is useful in the recovery period, because it contains substances that help in digestion and elimination.

OVERCOMING CONSTIPATION

What goes in at one end has to come out at the other! The diet of people who are confined to bed needs to be carefully balanced if they are not eliminating waste regularly. This is why fruit and vegetables and lots to drink are important. Just having a slight fever can make a person constipated, because the heat of the fever dehydrates the tubes. If all your efforts don't produce results, then help is needed.

Dried fruit such as dates, figs or prunes help some people. These can be stewed with apples, or puréed with apple or prune juice as a compôte, thus making a medicinal meal. Chickweed, in a salad or in a soup, root ginger, fresh and sliced very thin across the grain and infused, makes a tangy and pleasant 'tea'; the root can also be grated finely over either fresh fruit or a salad. Stewed rhubarb seldom fails, but linseed — one tablespoon simmered in half a pint of water and the lot taken like soup, perhaps flavoured with a pinch of fresh parsley — might appeal better to someone with a savoury preference.

If all else fails, use abdominal massage. The ileo-caecal valve is where the small intestine meets the large intestine, or colon. It's a non-return valve and is right beside your appendix (if you haven't had it removed). In 999 people out of 1,000, it's in the lower right quarter of the abdomen. The colon is a flexible tube with a many-pocketed wall. The pockets are designed to increase its surface area without increasing the width of the lumen, or 'bore'. Its main function is to absorb water out of the material that passes through it and to help that substance on its way. Lying in bed slows down the activity of the colon. Walking about hastens it on.

If someone is unable to walk and has not had recent abdominal surgery, start by pressing and kneading in that lower right quarter and work up toward the ribs, then across the abdomen from right to left just below the ribs and then down the left side of the abdomen as far as can be reached toward the inguinal groove — that's the inner fold of the hinge between the belly and the thigh. This can be done repeatedly and it can be done by the one who is constipated if the carer is otherwise occupied (including if he or she is having a quick nap!). If the sufferer is bed-bound, be sure a bedpan or a potty is close by, because the urge to pass may come on sudden and strong!

Hygiene

If a bedpan or a potty is available in the bedroom and the carer is not on hand to take it away as soon as it is used, be sure to have a cover there — even a folded newspaper is better than nothing. If a small amount of water with a couple of drops of a favourite essential oil is left in the vessel in preparation for its use, it both makes it easier to empty and also pleasanter to share the room with. Also, always leave a bowl of water, some soap and a towel for the sufferer to wash their hands with after they've used this improvised lavatory.

I keep emphasising washing the hands, because it is with our hands that we stroke our hair, pat dogs and cats and favoured children, wipe our bottoms, eat our food, etc., and thereby transmit the germs we have picked up. (On the Indian continent, people seldom use cutlery to eat with. They use the right hand because they have been taught that the left hand is reserved for washing, or wiping the bottom after elimination. All restaurants there have a source of clean water for their customers to wash their hands both before *and* after eating.)

DOCTOR'S VISITS

When the doctor calls, unless the sick person is a child under about ten years old, or very nervous, or for some reason unable to speak, leave the room and quietly shut the door. This prevents anyone getting embarrassed about asking for privacy and inspires confidence. You, as carer, can have your conversation with the doctor — also in privacy! — before he or she leaves the house.

VENTILATION

Ventilation is important in the bedroom. It is better for the air to be a bit cool but well circulated than warm and static. Anyone in bed can have an extra blanket for warmth. The risk is a draught, but there again, anyone in bed can be well wrapped up if there's any risk of a draught.

OTHER INCIDENTALS

Always make sure there are plenty of handkerchiefs, either paper or cloth close to the bed, also toys or books that the sufferer might want. Flowers are cheering and beneficial, but they don't need to be right by the bed. The carer may spend a lot of time reading aloud. In so far as is compatible with a healthy recovery, respect the wishes of the sufferer. If the sufferer is asleep, wake them only if the doctor calls and requests to see them awake, or if the house is burning down! Sleep is a great healer. Meals can wait and so can unsolicited telephone calls, or visitors.

CHAPTER EIGHT

The Tools and the Raw Materials

The tools used for making, and the containers used for storing, medicinal preparations should be only those that are as inert as possible. To heat preparations, earthenware is the traditional pan used by herbalists the world over, but fire-proof earthenware is very difficult to buy in the British Isles. Next best is fire-proof glass, or what today is called ceramic. Enamel is a form of glass — glass in powder form is fired onto a metal base to form a smooth, glazed surface. Provided this is unchipped, so none of the metal base is exposed, this is a good inert substance for the container. If you can afford to, it is wise to keep these containers and pans exclusively for preparing medicinal mixtures.

STERILISING CONTAINERS

Once the medication is prepared, glass jars or bottles make the best storage containers. These should be sterile when filled. There are two ways to do this. If you have ever made jam, pickles, wine or chutney, you will probably be familiar with the two ways of sterilising glass — the dry and wet methods. For the dry method, remove the lids and put the jars or bottles into the oven while it is still cold. Turn the heat on to 350°F–400°F/190°C/Gas Mark 5. Once the oven has reached that heat, maintain it for half an hour before turning it off. The jars or bottles may be removed hot, or left in the oven to cool, when their tops (screw tops, for preference) should be put on to maintain the sterility. Metal screw tops for jars and bottles often have a plastic lining — if the dry method is used to sterilise them, the plastic will distort. It is better to use the wet method only to sterilise lids.

For the wet method, use a large pan filled with cold water into which you submerge the glass containers, allowing them to fill as you do so. Bring this to the boil, and keep the water boiling fast for twenty minutes. At this point the jars, or bottles, may be removed individually while the water is still maintained at the boil and the jars are filled as they are removed (this is required in some recipes). Otherwise, the containers may be lifted out of the boiling water, placed upside down to drain and cool, after which the lids — which should also have been boiled — should be put on, if the containers are not to be used immediately.

How to Store Preparations

I advocate collecting glass containers of all sizes, provided they have good sealing lids and hoarding them until you need them. This way you are never at a loss for a container and you are recycling good glass at the same time. Some recipes, especially older ones, call for amber glass bottles. It is possible to buy these in a variety of sizes from pharmacies and from wholesalers. The amber tint in the glass protects the contents from ultraviolet light, which destroys the colour of herbs and may also leach out some of the beneficial qualities. It is not necessary to go to the expense of buying such amber glass if the preparation you are making can be stored in the fridge, however. The light in the fridge is not ultraviolet and the little man turns it off once you shut the door anyway!

If you intend to use a dark cupboard for storage, that's all right too. If you are going to use an exposed shelf, you can cover ordinary, clear glass with brown paper sleeves as protection. Never store any herbs or herbal preparations near heat or in direct sunlight, even if the containers are amber or protected with brown paper.

WATER

I have discussed the depleted quality of nourishment in commercially produced food. Mains supplied water is no better. At best it is dead, at worst, it may be dangerous. It contains so-called 'safe' levels of chemicals added to destroy harmful bacteria. It may also contain social medications such as fluorides. Some people are allergic to the substances added, legally, to tap water. Others simply dislike the smell or the taste.

It is important to use only uncontaminated water in your medicinal preparations. If you are unable to use fresh, spring water, drawn from a well by you, or someone you know, then the bottled variety — but not the carbonated sort, only still — is a fairly good substitute. If this is obtainable only in plastic rather than glass bottles, you may have to use distilled water, again in glass rather than plastic bottles, although distilled water is also dead.

If you think you live in an area where there should be a spring or a well but you can't find out where, try your local library for the name and address of a member of the British — or Irish — Association of Dowsers (see 'Helpful Addresses', page 117). A dowser can find a well for you, if one exists, and tell you if the water is potable — that means pure and drinkable. He or she may ask you to provide a map, either by the Ordnance Survey, or one you've drawn yourself. Don't be surprised if the dowser uses a pendulum over your map to find the source of water! It sounds like magic, but it's surprisingly accurate.

OILS

It's better for the quality of the remedies you intend to make to begin with the best of everything. Water is the base for a large range of preparations and oil is the base for many others. Organic oils will give the best results, whether they are used for massage or as an ingredient in a lotion, an ointment or a poultice. Infusions of oil are also called medicated or fixed oils. If you intend to make your own, which is easy to do, you need a good organic oil. The choice is olive, sunflower, safflower or almond. Avoid soya oil because it goes rancid very easily, although a few drops of wheatgerm oil added to any other oil will retard the oxidation process that causes rancidity.

A store of unpainted glass beads can take the place of the little marbles pharmacists of long ago used to pour into bottles and jars to replace liquid they had removed and to bring the surface of the contents to the top of the neck of the container to exclude the air. If you do this, remember to sterilise the beads or marbles and to keep them in a sterile container until you use them. You can buy oils as above and also ready-prepared fixed oils from reputable wholesalers, some of which are listed in 'Helpful Addresses', pages 117–18.

Essential oils — lavender, rose, juniper, etc. — require complicated processes for their extraction. This is best left to the expert who has the resources for the expensive equipment needed. Some oils, such as rose or sandalwood, either take vast quantities of petals, or are from rare and exotic woods and so are very costly to produce. These are sometimes diluted by other oils to bring the price down and make the oil accessible to more people. Reputable suppliers will label the oil appropriately, for example, Rose in Jojoba. Dilute oils of this sort are used in just the same way as non-diluted essential oils.

FATS

Animal fats are used in ointments and creams that require a good absorption factor. Unbleached petroleum jelly — Vaseline — makes a protective rather than an absorbent preparation. Of the animal fats, the most common to be used are lard, goose-grease and ghee, or refined butter (much favoured by Ayurvedic herbalists).

When making your choice of fats, try to remember two important factors: that the source is organic, so that no traces of undesirable chemicals are included and that no one using a preparation that includes any of these fats is allergic to them. People allergic to milk products, for example, will be allergic to ghee. Those allergic to pork will be allergic to lard, as lard is made by heating the belly section of a pig's carcass until the soft fat runs out. (Dripping is another animal fat, made in the same way but from suet, the fat surrounding the kidneys of cattle, sheep or goats. It sets much harder than lard and was used to make candles and tapers in years gone by.) Lard is usually then separated from any fibrous or fleshy parts by straining and added to water and boiled, before cooling. When cooled, it will have separated from the water, and any impurities are at the part in contact with the water on which it floats.

If you buy lard in packets, there will be a statement on the wrapper that it contains 'permitted antioxidant', but this substance is not identified. Regard it as a pollutant and make your own, or obtain it from a trustworthy friend who can make it for you.

Goose-grease runs out of a goose as it's roasting. If

you cook one of these birds, beware — it contains much more fat than you ever believed!

Ghee is made from unsalted butter which is heated in an appropriate pan, such as those listed at the beginning of this chapter. Use a low flame. When the butter boils, reduce the heat still further. After the butter has become a clear golden yellow, it will start to smell like popcorn. At this stage it should be free from water. To test if it is water-free, drop a tiny quantity of water into the boiling butter. If it spits and crackles, all the water has gone. Wait until the sound has stopped and then take the pan away from the heat and allow the contents to stand for a few minutes.

Strain it while still hot into hot, wide-necked jars and secure the lids. If you pour the hot fat into cold jars, you run the risk of cracking them, just as if you pour cold liquid into hot jars the same thing can happen. Ghee will keep for up to a year without going rancid, unlike untreated butter.

ALCOHOL

Alcohol is used as an extractive agent in the preparation of tinctures and, again, you need only the best. Even the most expensive brandies, vodkas and whiskeys are only second best, I believe. Unless you're prepared to use illicit distillations, however, such as poteen — made by a reputable, if outlawed, distiller — you cannot be sure of no additives. No matter how pure a commercial alcohol is, it will contain something to alter the colour, or the specific gravity, or something else.

SYRUPS

When you're making syrup, it's the sugar or honey you use that causes the syrup to thicken. Here again, it's important to use the best available. Whether to use sugar or honey is your personal choice. If you choose sugar, unrefined organically grown is what you need — made from cane, not from beet. I've never seen a recipe for a syrup made from black-strap molasses, but in theory it should be possible. Molasses is rich in iron and other minerals that are very beneficial to people who are run down, or anaemic.

Honey should be unmixed, unboiled and as near its natural state as possible, but in this instance it is best to use honey that has been extracted from the comb. It doesn't matter if the honey is clear or granulated. The heating process will de-granulate it. Some honey is emulsified, or homogenised, which makes it look opaque but smooth, and it never granulates. My reaction to this is to be suspicious of it, because I don't know how it is achieved and in any case it has always seemed to me unnecessary to interfere with honey, because in its natural state it is totally pure and will keep indefinitely.

BEESWAX

Beeswax is required for ointments and lotions. If you don't keep bees, their wax can be bought from wholefood shops, or pharmacies. Pharmacies are more likely to stock bleached beeswax (its natural colour is a yellowy-beige), often shaped into little pearls, rather than the usual one-ounce blocks. If you have no choice, buy what you can get. Bleaching is the nearest to being messed about that beeswax can get.

It is up to you to ensure that the herbs you use to make medications are the best obtainable, either by your own gathering, or from reputable commercial sources. 'Helpful Addresses' has some addresses you may find useful.

CHAPTER NINE

Definitions, Recipes and a Few Formulae

DEFINITIONS OF MEDICAL TERMS

Analgesia = pain remover

Anthelmintic = Vermifuge = expels intestinal worms

Aperient = Laxative = Purgative = induces bowel action

Astringent = contracts tissue

Cardiac = of the heart

Carminative = relieves flatulence

Demulcent = loosens or removes phlegm or mucous

Diaphoretic = promotes perspiration

Diuretic = induces urination

Emetic = induces vomiting

Emollient = softening and soothing

Emmenagogue = promotes menstruation

Febrifuge = breaks a fever

Formula = medical recipe

Homeostasis = normal function

Mydriatic = causes dilation of the pupil of the eye

Myotic = causes contraction of the pupil of the eye

Nephritic = Renal = of kidney

Nervine = restores nerves

Oxytocic = stimulates uterine contractions

Pectoral = of chest or lungs

Psyche = mind

Pulmonary = of the lungs

Pyretic = prevents fever

Simple = medicament from a single substance

Soma = body

Soporific = sleep inducing

Styptic = coagulates blood

BASIC RECIPES AND FORMULAE

BATHS

There are four kinds of remedial bath:

- for hands, wrists or elbows
- for feet or ankles
- for lower torso immersion (a sitting, or sitz, bath)
- a whole body bath.

In a whole body bath, it is usually recommended that the area over and above the heart is kept out of the water — in other words, submerge the body as far as the lower ribs only. A bath is usually taken in hot water, but not so hot as to make the flesh go red, and lasts for fifteen to twenty minutes. The water has added to it a tincture, an infusion, or a few drops of an essential oil, thus medicating it. Usually, on ending the bath, the flesh that has been immersed is allowed to dry at room temperature, not rinsed or wiped. After a whole body bath, it is often recommended to wrap the body in a warm towel and, covered with blankets, for the person to sleep for as long as possible.

Basins or buckets are suitable for bathing hands, feet, ankles and elbows.

Bathing the hands or the feet can have a profound effect on the internal organs. A headache, or a chill in the kidneys, can be relieved by bathing the feet in an appropriate bath. This is because the energies of the body change polarity at the four extremities where they are at their most volatile and receptive. Bathing the feet can affect the spleen, liver, stomach, gall-bladder, urinary bladder and the kidneys. Bathing the hands can affect the lungs, colon, heart, small intestines and body-fluids. Which

organ(s) is/are affected depends on the choice of
medication added to the bath.

Some baths use the actual material, not a previously
prepared medicated liquid. Examples are oat baths. Both
grain and straw can be used, or sea-vegetables such as kelp
or bladderwrack. Pre-heated, these are added to the water
in the bath. (Sea vegetables retain heat better than other
substances.)

COMPRESS

A compress is a piece of cloth, a towel or a swab that has
been saturated with an infusion, a decoction, a diluted
tincture or water to which a few drops of an essential oil
has been added. A compress can also be a piece of cloth
etc. that has been saturated simply with hot or cold water.

A medicated compress is usually applied warm, rather
than hot or cold and is covered by dry cloth and perhaps a
piece of plastic to keep the moisture in near the skin. This
is especially necessary if the person to whom the compress
is being applied is to stay in bed, or to sleep the night with
it on.

CREAM (OR LOTION)

This is my preferred recipe from the several possible
options.

Ingredients 1

    16 parts medicated oil
     8 parts tincture, decoction or infusion
     4 parts good beeswax
     4 parts animal fat, or vegetable oil, or petroleum jelly
    ¼ part powdered borax (as well as being an
        emulsifier, borax has a soothing quality of its own)

The following ingredients can be adapted for cosmetic use
as well.

Ingredients 2

> 1 litre/36 fl oz Almond oil, plus 2.5 ml/30 drops
> Rose Absolute added
> 0.5 litre/18 fl oz Rose water
> 250 g/10 oz beeswax
> 250 g/10 oz ghee (if hands are chapped, for instance)
> *or* 250 g/10 oz petroleum jelly (if protection is
> sought, only)
> 15 g/½ oz powdered borax

Method

The method is the same for either of the above sets of ingredients.

Use a double saucepan (enamel), or a basin standing on a plinth in a pan of boiling water. The plinth can be a shallow tin with one end removed and holes stabbed in the other, e.g. a tin that once held fish. It would double as a pastry cutter. This will prevent the bottom of the basin from coming into contact with the bottom of the pan.

In this vessel, gently heat the beeswax and the 4 parts animal fat (or petroleum jelly). In a separate vessel, similar to the first, gently heat the 16 parts medicated oil. Once the beeswax has melted, add the warm oil to that pan.

Finally, in a third vessel, heat the tincture, decoction, infusion, or Rose water and dissolve the borax powder in it.

Now comes the bit that resembles the making of real mayonnaise. Very slowly — and stirring continually — pour the borax solution into the wax/oil mixture, which is still on a gentle heat. Once all is combined, remove from the heat and continue to stir until the mixture is cold. If you stop stirring for more than a few moments, the mixture can separate irrevocably and will require re-heating and stirring continually, yet again.

When cold and totally emulsified, pour into wide-necked glass jars.

DECOCTION

A decoction is what you are doing whenever you percolate, or simmer, real ground coffee. An infusion is not sufficiently vigorous to extract the virtue from the harder parts of plants, roots, twigs, barks and larger or harder seeds. Decocting involves boiling these plant parts in water for the prescribed amount of time, which may vary from recipe to recipe. Proportions of plant material to water are similar to those for an infusion (see below). When the remedy is ready to bottle, it should be strained, not filtered, because some sediment is desirable.

A decoction, bottled into sterile bottles and capped tight, will keep for about one month, in the fridge. If small white blobs appear on the surface of the remedy, it has started to decompose and should be given to the compost heap whence it will benefit you in some other way!

INFUSION

An infusion is what you are making every time you brew a cup of tea! A standard remedial infusion is 25 g/1 oz dried (or 50 g/2 oz fresh) herb — leaf or flower or small seeds, such as fennel or celery — to 600 ml/1 pt boiling water. This amount makes a strong infusion, representing a course of doses over one, or possibly two, days. An infusion is for short-term use.

Dosing may be in spoonfuls, glasses or cups, whatever the recommendation of the specific remedy. When drunk, the infusion should be diluted with an equal amount of hot water so that it is taken warm, unless otherwise stated.

INHALATIONS

These are used for the upper respiratory system and facial sinuses, or for the urinary or vaginal areas. In either case, a basin or small bowl containing very hot water to which a volatile, remedial oil has been added, is placed conveniently. The bowl and the head, or the lower body as appropriate, is wrapped in towels to retain the steam, which is the remedial agent. Breathe in through the nose and out through the mouth. 'Wink' the lower parts by contracting and relaxing the muscles of the pelvic floor in succession.

If inhalations for the lower body are likely to be needed over a long period, it may be worthwhile acquiring — or improvising — a commode, which is a chair with a basin let into the seat, usually with a hinged lid over it.

MEDICATED OIL

Using any of the oils listed in the previous chapter, fill a wide-necked glass jar with fresh herb, broken as small as possible. (There is a school of thought that believes it is injurious to use any metal containing iron to cut herbal material for medicinal purposes, hence breaking rather than cutting.) Once the jar is as full as possible, cover the contents with your chosen oil. Secure the lid of the jar.

Stand the jar either in a sunny place or somewhere warm, such as the airing cupboard or the overmantle of the range. Give it a good shake at least once a day for fourteen days. If you stand the jar in the sun, cover it with a black cloth or a brown paper sleeve to protect the colour of the herbs. The fourteen days is recommended as from the full of the moon to the dark of the moon, when the oil should be strained, but not filtered. Store out of direct light.

OINTMENT

You can make an ointment by adapting the cream/lotion formula as above. By changing the proportions, but retaining the overall weight/quantity, it is possible to make something that will set harder:

Ingredients

Reduce the 16 parts medicated oil to 12 parts
Increase the beeswax to 6 parts
Increase the animal fat/petroleum jelly to 6 parts

Method

Proceed with the method as for the cream/lotion.

There is an alternative formula, and two methods for preparing it.

Ingredients

To 1 part finely crumbled dried herb
or 2 parts finely broken fresh herb
add 3 parts animal fat, *or* petroleum jelly, *or* vegetable oil

Method 1

Using a double saucepan, or the same improvisation suggested for the lotion, put all the ingredients into the upper part of the vessel. Without allowing the water in the lower part of the vessel to boil fast, and stirring occasionally, leave this on a low heat for 3–4 hours.
At the end of this time, strain any lumpiness out of the mixture by passing it through a jelly bag, or a piece of coarse cotton or linen cloth. If you have used finely pulverised or powdered herbs, there's no need to strain the ointment, but the herbal content may shorten its shelf life.

Method 2

Place all the ingredients in a heavy enamel or earthenware casserole with a close fitting lid. Put this in the bottom of the oven (this is an ideal method for people with ranges) at a low temperature — a very slow oven, around 225°/110°C/Gas Mark ¼, and leave for 6–8 hours. Overnight will do fine. After this time, follow the directions for straining as given above in Method 1.

POULTICE

A poultice is made from the material parts of a herb, or some other substance through which herbs or herb extracts, e.g. an infusion, have been mixed.

Finely chop, mince, break or liquidise the material intended for use. Add a small amount of comb honey to it if you want it to cohere better, or if an additional anti-bacterial quality is required of the dressing. Spread the material on a single thickness of cotton or linen cloth — a man's handkerchief, or a fragment of an old sheet is ideal. (To use man-made fibre is not a good idea, because it can irritate the skin and prevent sufficient movement of moisture between the plant material and the skin.) Allow a depth of about 1.2 cm/½ in and an area slightly larger than the area the poultice is intended to cover. Fold the edges of the cloth over the herbal material until it is completely covered.

Apply the poultice to the affected area with the single thickness of cloth next to the skin and the folded edges of the cloth outermost. Keep it in place with non-stretchy sticky plaster, or a broad, soft bandage. Usually a poultice is intended to remain in place for a minimum of twelve hours — for example, all night, or for twenty-four hours. For a very small poultice, such as a folded ivy leaf to cover a corn, no cloth is required as a wrapping, just some plaster to keep it in place.

SYRUP

Syrup is usually made from a decoction of, say, fruit such as rose-hips or elderberries, or from flowers. First make the decoction, boiling well to extract all the virtue from the plant material. Strain the decoction. Then to every 600 ml/1 pt of liquid add 500g/1 lb of cane sugar, or pure, unmixed, unboiled, natural honey. Return to the boil, stirring constantly, and allow to boil fast for one minute, still stirring. Bottle immediately into hot bottles. Cap and store in the fridge, or on a shelf in a cool, dry place.

TINCTURE

This is a way of preserving the virtues of a plant almost indefinitely. It is not a straightforward alternative either to an infusion or a decoction for two reasons. Because it uses alcohol, it extracts substances water alone cannot extract — resins and oils for example. It is used in smaller doses than either infusions or decoctions and it works with the energies of the body to a greater degree than either of these, but also at the physical level.

A tincture is made as follows. Fill a wide-necked jar with the fresh herbs of your choice. Fresh herbs are better than dried, because some virtue can be lost in the drying process. Cover the broken herbs (see 'Medicated Oil', page 71, for why to break rather than cut) with either pure alcohol, or a mixture of around fifty per cent pure water to fifty per cent pure alcohol. By 'pure', I mean good quality brandy or whiskey, or — preferably — vodka or home distilled alcohol. An organic wine or cider vinegar can be used instead, but this should not be diluted with water. Stand the jar in a warm place — as for a medicated oil — shaking several times a day for the fourteen days between the full and the dark of the moon. Strain rather than filter into sterile bottles. Cap and store in a cool dry place, out of direct light.

EXTRA TIPS

Whatever you make, always label the filled containers, detailing the name of the formula/simple, the form — decoction, or tincture, etc. — and the date of making, before you put it into store, or out for use! Do not deep-freeze any part of your medications at any stage and always store them out of the reach of children — not all of them will do them any harm, but how frustrating if one devoured all your elder-syrup!

APPLICATIONS AND DOSAGES

Preparations using water are direct in their absorption of the physiological energies of the plant. They are most suited, when used internally, to warm weather and acute symptoms. Alcohol, as used in the preparation of tinctures, absorbs different components of plant material. In other words, water soluble parts of plants are not necessarily alcohol soluble, and vice versa. The energetics of tinctures are often more subtle than infusions or decoctions and are more suited to cold weather and chronic conditions.

Some individuals respond better to water-based preparations than alcohol or oil-based ones and the other way round is equally true. Sometimes the tincture will treat the opposite problem from that treated by the infusion or decoction. Experience and books with more detail will be needed for more information on this subject.

BASIC RULES

These are subject to variation by the judgment of the
herbalist:

> Internal dosage: up to 3 times a day
> Infusion/Decoction: 10 g/¼ oz per dose,
>> (i.e. 30 g/ 1 oz per day)
> Alcohol-based Tincture: 50–100 drops per dose
>> (up to 300 per day)
> Essential oil: 3 drops per dose (9 drops per day)
> External applications: compresses, usually dilute as for
>> internal use
> Poultices: not more than twice a day, but left on for
>> duration, i.e. 12 or 24 hours. Longer than 24
>> hours is inadvisable.

Large people need larger doses. Children (small people)
need smaller doses. Doses given above relate to medium
sized adults. Scale up or down, as appropriate.

FLOWER ESSENCES AS REMEDIES

Flower remedies work equally well to adjust emotional
and mental problems, as well as some physical ones. The
best known are Dr Bach's thirty-eight flower essences and
his combination, Rescue Remedy. His range is made by
two producers in the UK, both listed in 'Helpful
Addresses', page 117. Books about this range of herbal-
based remedies are listed in 'Recommended Reading',
pages 119–20.

The making of flower remedies is, at a practical level, a
bit similar to making an infusion or a tincture, but is very
mindful of the site and condition of the source plants, the
time of day and the weather conditions as well as the
spiritual focus of the maker. To this end, flower remedies
represent a bridge between the herbal/esoteric medicine
of Aboriginal practitioners and the materialist/herbal

practices of European origin. There are two methods, one or other more appropriate to the type of flower you choose to make into an essence. You are not restricted to the range chosen by Dr Edward Bach and many other ranges have been developed in recent years; they all incorporate the esoteric as well as the herbal source of healing.

THE SUN METHOD

Choose a site where the flowers (one species at a time) grow naturally and freely away from any of the potential contaminants listed in 'Where To Pick', pages 30–31. Choose a bright, sunny day that looks pretty settled. You need the following tools and additional substances:

- a thin, undecorated glass bowl (not fire-proof), about the size of a cereal bowl
- a glass jug
- a glass funnel
- 2 bottles with screw tops, one of about 300 ml/ ½ pt, the other of about 600 ml/1 pt
- equal volume of good alcohol (brandy is what is used in the commercially made essences) and fresh well, or spring, water. Do *not* use distilled or tap water.

Between 8–9 a.m. in the morning, take your bowl to the plant site. Fill the bowl with the water you have brought with you in the smaller of the two bottles — set the bottle aside carefully and with its lid on, because you are going to need it again. Pick, where possible, flowers on stalks and either shake them onto the surface of the water, or ease them off with a twig or stalk from the same plant. Don't touch the flowers with your fingers and — especially important — from the time you fill the glass bowl with water, let no shadow — your own, other plants, other creatures, or clouds — pass across the surface of the water. If this happens, abandon the process and start again on another day.

Once the surface of the water has been covered with flowers, all at peak condition and from as many plants as possible in that colony of the plants you have chosen, allow the bowl to sit in the sun where it is. You should have all the preparation completed by shortly after 9 a.m. Stay near the bowl as a guardian to protect it from the shadows of creatures and focus on the energy of the sun which is transferring the energies of the flowers to the water.

Water is an amazing substance, about which whole books have been written and of which more should be generally known! The water will be potentised by the sunlit flower energy. You may stop the process at around noon, after which the sun's energy will begin to wane, having allowed plus or minus three hours, according to your intuition.

The flowers should be removed from the surface of the water using more stalks, or twigs, from the same plants. Once the surface is clear, you may decant the water into the jug and pour it carefully into the bottle again. At the site, or at home — in any case as soon as possible — blend this potentised water with an equal volume of alcohol in the larger bottle. At all times treat the bottle of potentised water as though it is the most precious thing you have ever handled. Treat the alcohol/water mix in the same way, — this is the mother bottle.

To a 30 ml/1 oz bottle, with a dropper in and filled with alcohol, add two drops from the mother bottle. This is your stock bottle. From the stock bottle you take drops into dose bottles. The dose bottle should also be 30 ml/ 1 oz and have a dropper. It can be filled with spring/well water and to it drops are added from the selection of remedies that are chosen. The number of drops depends on the choice of the practitioner — you can be your own practitioner, because flower essences can be safely used by untrained people and were thus intended by Dr Bach.

THE BOILING METHOD

This also requires a good day for the selection of the flowers. Again you take the vessel to the site, but this time it should be an earthenware or an enamel pan. Into it you place the flowers, using the same method as outlined above for the sun method. When the pan is about three-quarters full of flowers, with stalks no more than about 3.7 cm/ 1½ in long, put on the lid and carry it with great care and reverence to the house. Once there, the flowers should be covered with clean well or spring water, up to about 300 ml/½ pt.

Without the lid on, bring the pan to the boil and simmer for half an hour. If the flowers need to be immersed during this simmering time, use a twig to push them down again — a twig of the same plant. Replace the lid when the cooking time is over and leave the pan outside to cool. When cold, the essence should be filtered. Filter paper is the only additional thing you will require. As before, your fingers should not come into contact with the flowers or the water in which they have been simmered.

After filtering the essence and cooling it, combine it with the same volume of alcohol as you have essence. From here, follow the directions as for the sun method.

These preparation techniques are paraphrased — with his permission — from Julian Barnard's book, *The Healing Herbs of Dr Bach*. This is an area of herbal medicine that is growing in application and, I believe, should be better known. It is, like the more conventional herbalism, accessible to all, without any special training.

CHAPTER TEN

Formulae and Specific Problems

Although western culture in general, both religious and philosophic, seeks to deny the individual a personal expression of any spirituality they may feel, there are many people who are aware of an energy that comes from some deep connection with a source beyond themselves. People interpret it in different ways and have their own personal names for it. If it feels right to you, I urge you to give in to this and to use whatever feels right to you as an intended thought form of love, goodwill, harmony, or however you experience it. Use this especially in the preparing of food and, of course, remedies. It makes a real difference. Don't listen to the news bulletin as you do it, as that form of negativity is damaging.

On the whole, I have always found the simples work best in whatever appropriate form. Most of the things you are called on to treat are not complicated anyway, so a simple works best. However, I have both devised and adapted some formulae, as follows.

JOOD'S JOLLOP

This is an endlessly useful formula I created over twenty years ago. It was the first formula I invented for myself and it has broad application as a demulcent, or phlegm/mucous shifter, for people of all ages. It got its name from my family. It works for catarrh whether it's stuffing up the sinuses in the way that gives those horrible, congested headaches, or choking the airways after a cold, or for people with chronic bronchitis who can't hawk up the phlegm in their bronchial tubes, or indeed for mucous that's clogging any bodily part.

INGREDIENTS

25 g/1 oz each of the following dried herbs:
Coltsfoot leaves
Thyme leaves
Ground Fenugreek seed
800 ml/1½ pt cold spring water

METHOD

Add the herbs to the water in a double saucepan (enamel) and set to heat slowly. Stir the mixture from time to time, because the Fenugreek has a habit of sticking to the bottom of the pan. Simmer gently for about 2 hours, or until the mixture resembles greeny-brown sludge.

Then put 2 generous tablespoonfuls of good honey (not comb) into a quart jug, or a lipped basin, and strain the sludge into this through a moderate gauge sieve, persuading it with a wooden spoon. Very little residue should remain. Scrape the underside of the sieve to be sure all the sludge goes onto the honey. Stir well to ensure that the honey is well dissolved and amalgamated with the rest.

Into a 600 ml/1 pt glass bottle, pour 1 fl oz/ 2 tablespoonfuls of good whiskey. Swill this round the bottle, which will doubly ensure the bottle's sterility and then pour in the sludge/honey mixture. Cap it and shake it well.

DOSE

The dose is one dessertspoon not less than 5 times a day for adults and the same number of times, but a teaspoonful, for children under eight years old. Shake well before you use it — the alcohol tends to rise and the sludge to fall!

HERNIA POULTICE

The following is a formula I have used recently for my husband's hernia. It was given to me by a friend — a qualified western pharmacist before he trained in Chinese medicine — who practises Chinese medicine using acupuncture and Chinese herbs. This formula is intended to strengthen and rejuvenate the slack tissues that cause the hernia, which is in the lower right quadrant of the abdomen. This is the formula, but, as you'll see, it takes more than mere materials.

INGREDIENTS

Dried, powdered Bentonite clay (available from a craft potter's supplier)
Tincture of Comfrey *(Symphytum)*
Tincture of Marigold *(Calendula)*
The tinctures you can have either bought or made.

METHOD

Measure out a volume of the Bentonite powder that you estimate to be sufficient to cover generously the swollen area of the hernia to a depth of about three-quarters of an inch. Measure out an equal volume of spring water and add this to the Bentonite. To this add ⅕ of the volume of the water of each of the tinctures; for example, if you have used 50 cc of clay and 50 cc of water, you need 10 cc of Comfrey tincture and 10 cc of Marigold tincture. Mix this with a wooden or bone tool until all the moisture is absorbed into the clay.

At this point, take a ball of the mix in your hand, having divided it into roughly equal parts, each lump fitting comfortably into the palm of your hand. It should feel like soft plasticine. Focus your mind on the healing energy of the plants and of the volcanic dust, which is the Bentonite and on the energy that brought it out of the bowels of the earth. Feel the energy of your hands enhancing the plant and clay energy. As you focus in this way, knead each lump of clay. Once you are satisfied that each lump is well worked and well energised — there is no time-limit, just when you feel it to be so — set that lump aside and start on the next one, in the same way.

Eventually, amalgamate all the lumps and shape the single piece to fit over the hernia. I use a plastic sheet over the poultice to prevent it drying out or staining clothes, and tie it into place with a silk scarf that I knot over my husband's hip. He looks quite rakish! He sleeps with this in place, removing it in the morning.

SCAR TISSUE POULTICE

There's another poultice formula as follows, that is useful for scar tissue, whether from accident or surgery.

INGREDIENTS

Slippery Elm powder
Comfrey root, peeled and liquidised

METHOD

Use equal volumes of the Slippery Elm powder and Comfrey root. Work the ingredients into a paste. Use the same focus of attention as for the Bentonite poultice.

This poultice can be used at any time after all scabs have cleared from the wound — even old scars have been known to respond to it. Apply the paste liberally all over the scar area and bind into place in whatever way is appropriate.

Note: Slippery Elm powder is quite distinct from Slippery Elm food, which is cut with flour and other things. For all medicinal purposes, it is Slippery Elm powder that is required.

IMMUNE SYSTEM AND ESSIAC

In the section on Cancer in Chapter Six I mentioned Essiac. This formula works wonders for a depleted immune system, whatever disorder is the result of this depletion.

Essiac does three things: it cleans the blood, cleans the liver and oxygenates the cells. As a result of taking it, a sick person feels more energetic and has a greater sense of well-being. The formula originated among the Ojibwe people of North America, one of whom gave it to a white woman about the turn of the last century. She in her turn gave it to a highly qualified and experienced nurse in an Ontario hospital in 1922. The name of the nurse was Rene Caisse, who for some reason chose to reverse her surname to make a name for the formula.

Many romantic stories have grown up around the use of Essiac and numerous 'cures' are linked to it. I know personally many people who have benefited enormously from using it, and who have baffled their doctors by overturning their prognoses. An improved quality of life, including the minimising of pain, has also been recorded by people whose loved ones have died while taking Essiac, when their condition has been too far gone for reversal. Before you get carried away with the idea of Essiac as a miracle cure, please remember that no remedy, whatever it is, works one hundred per cent for everybody.

The mystical number 4 figures large in the philosophy of the Ojibwe and this is reflected in the formula.

INGREDIENTS

Burdock, root *(Arctium lappa)*
Sheep Sorrel, leaf *(Rumex acetosella)*
Slippery Elm, powder *(Ulvus fulma)*
Turkey Rhubarb, root powder *(Rheum officinale)*

The proportions of these 4 ingredients are in multiples of 4:

    24 parts Burdock root
    16 parts Sheep Sorrel
     4 parts Slippery Elm
     1 part Turkey Rhubarb

METHOD

Add 100 g/4 oz of the formula, in the above proportions
of the 4 dried ingredients, to 5 litres/8 pt of spring water
once the water has reached a rolling boil. Use a 10 litre/
2-gallon vessel to boil this in for 12 minutes. Check that
all the herbs are submerged in the liquid; replace the lid
and leave the decoction to steep for a minimum of
6 hours (all night is ideal). Then remove the lid again, and
give it a good stir. Replace the lid and leave to steep for a
further minimum of 6 hours.

Re-heat. Strain into sterile, hot bottles, label and use.
The average shelf life is about a month.

DOSE

The dose is 4 tablespoonfuls diluted with an equal amount
of boiling spring water. To be most effective, this dose
should be taken on a fasting stomach — 2 hours before
the dose without any food or drink and one hour after.
For someone who is really ill, 3 doses a day may be taken
— this is the maximum that should be taken. Try waking,
taking the first dose and waiting one hour for breakfast.
Have lunch at, say, 1 p.m. You will have finished eating by
1.30 p.m., so eat or drink nothing until 3.30 p.m., when
you take the second dose. Wait another hour and at
4.30 p.m. you can have tea, if you feel like it. When you
have decided what time you want to go to bed, take no
food or drink for 2 hours before that time, then take your
last dose of the day and go to bed.

EFFECT OF TAKING ESSIAC

After 6 to 8 weeks of taking Essiac 3 times a day, it will be
possible to see distinct changes in your state of health.
Some people find that changes happen quickly, others that
they happen more slowly. Don't be either despondent or
elated by this, because each person's system has its own

pace. Minimising of pain can happen within 3–4 days of starting to take this formula.

Once you feel sure there has been an improvement, cut out the dose in the middle of the day and take 2 doses a day for the next 3–4 months. After that, you may feel it is the right time to drop another dose. The evening dose may be the best one to retain, but you should make your own judgment, as you know your own body best. I suggest it merely because the blood pools in the liver when we lie down, so the work of the dose is simplified. Stay on one dose a day for about 6 months. A maintenance dose of, say, twice a week can then be taken. Some people take this formula as a prophylactic, one dose a day from the beginning.

DECOCTION FOR GENERAL USE

INGREDIENTS

50 g/2 oz Pot Barley (organic)

4 litre/5 pt spring water

2 oranges, or 2 lemons (organic, if possible)

100 g/4 oz glucose powder

METHOD

Simmer the barley and water until the barley is soft and the water reduced by half. If the fruits are not organic, wash them first, then peel them carefully and chop the flesh into the liquid. If organic fruit is used, it can be washed and sliced straight into the liquid. Stir in the glucose powder until it is dissolved.

Allow the decoction to steep for about 12 hours — perhaps all night. Squeeze out the pieces of citrus fruit and discard the skins. Bottle the decoction and use it as soon as possible, while it's still fresh.

Lemon — or orange — barley water is nourishing, soothing and refreshing, although the citrus in it may make it difficult to drink for people with mumps, measles, or chickenpox. If the sufferer doesn't like it, the carer can enjoy its qualities instead!

WEIGHTS AND MEASURES AND CONVERSIONS

APOTHECARY'S WEIGHT

(Different from Trading Weight, otherwise known as Avoirdupois.)

> 20 grains = 1 scruple
> 3 scruples = 1 drachm (or dram)
> 8 drachms = 1 ounce
> 12 ounces = 12 ounces = 1 pound = Troy weight,
>   (measure of precious metals)

APOTHECARY'S FLUID MEASURE

> 1 minim = 1 drop
> 60 drops = 1 drachm
> 8 drachms = 1 ounce
> 4 drachms = 1 tablespoon = 20 ml
> 2 ounces = 1 wineglassful
> 3 ounces = 1 teacupful
> 20 ounces = 1 pint
> 1.76 pints = 1 litre
> 8 pints = 1 gallon

SPECIFIC PROBLEMS — HOW TO TREAT THEM

When I had a sick person or an accident to deal with, I wanted to discover a book that listed problems and what helped them. So in this section I have listed problems in the following groups: Accidents, Disorders, Infections, Parasites and Female Reproduction. Under these headings are listed the herbs that are of benefit. These lists are far from comprehensive, but the herbs are common in the wild and can be cultivated or bought from suppliers (see 'Helpful Addresses', pages 117–18).

PREGNANCY

As pregnancy is a particularly special time for women, I have separated it out from the tables.

DIET

During pregnancy, it is good for both you and the growing baby if you eat nutritious foods, especially for the prevention and recovery from anaemia. Include the following in your diet:

- Alfalfa shoots
- Jerusalem Artichokes — steamed
- Asparagus — steamed
- Burdock root — steamed
- Chickweed — in salads and soups
- Chicory — in salads
- Comfrey leaf — in salads
- Dandelion — leaf and root
- Flower pollen — also known as bee pollen
- Carrageen (sea vegetable) — as a dessert, flavoured with three drops of orange or rose or lemon oil
- Nasturtium — leaves and flowers in salads and teas, seeds pickled
- Nettles — young and fresh as vegetable, dried as tea
- Red Clover — flowers in salads and teas
- Walnuts — as nuts, or pickled
- Watercress — in salads and soups

ACCIDENTS	THERAPEUTIC PLANTS	PLANT PART USED	FORM USED	METHOD
Burns	Aloe Vera	gel from inside leaf	as is	Cover entire area of burn with any one of these 4 remedies. Use liquid Five Flower or Rescue remedy internally as soon as burn occurs to arrival at casualty and beyond.
	Houseleek (*Sempervivum tectorum*)	as above	as above	
	Lavender (*Lavendula Officinalis*)	essential oil	neat	
	Rescue or Five Flower liquid and cream		as supplied	
Sprains	Comfrey (*Symphytum officinale*)	root	poultice or ointment	Ointment and crepe bandage useful by day, poultice and crepe bandage by night.
Thorns	Blackberry (*Rubus villosus*)	leaf	as is	Apply to site with underside of leaf to flesh; use sticking plaster to retain.
Broken Bones	Comfrey (*Symphytum officinale*)	root leaf	poultice infusion	Five Flower or Rescue at outset. Drink infusion regularly from first day. Use poultice after cast is removed.

ACCIDENTS	THERAPEUTIC PLANTS	PLANT PART USED	FORM USED	METHOD
Foreign bodies in the eye	Five Flower liquid or Rescue liquid		eye wash	*Always* dilute before using in eye. Direct wash with dropper. Wash eye from infusion — 2 teaspoons
	Eyebright (*Euphrasia officinalis*)	plant	infusion	herb in 1 cup boiling water. Cool to use as for Eyebright.
	Purple Loosestrife (*Lythrum salicaria*)	flowers and leaves	infusion	
DISORDERS				
Stomach acidity and indigestion	Horsetail (*Equisetum arvense*)	barren stem (after fruit)	ashes	3 to 10 grains between meals
Bunions	Ivy (*Hedera helix*)	leaf	tincture leaf	Soak leaves in cold apple cider vinegar for one week (or longer). Apply leaf to bunion, one per 24 hours, for 3 days. Repeat as necessary and wear *comfortable*, flat shoes.
Boils to draw	Periwinkle (*Vinca minor, or major*)	leaf	poultice	Chop leaves finely. Mix with comb honey. Apply thickly for 24 hours. Continue until effective.

DISORDERS	THERAPEUTIC PLANTS	PLANT PART USED	FORM USED	METHOD
Boils to drain	Comfrey (*Symphytum officinale*)	root	poultice	Chop, mince or liquidise cleaned root. Apply thick as poultice for 24 hours.
Boils to wash between dressings	Scarlet pimpernel (*Anagallis arvensis*)	plant	infusion or tincture	For all the following: full infusion or 5–10 drops of tincture in ½ cup warm water.
	Sage (*Salvia officinalis*)	leaf	infusion or tincture	As above
	St John's wort (*Hypericum perfoliatum*)	plant	as above	As above
	Tansy (*Tanacetum vulgare*)	plant	as above	As above
	Thyme (*Thymus vulgaris*)	plant	as above	As above
	Tormentil (*Potentilla tormentilla*)	plant	as above	As above
	Yarrow (*Achillea millefolium*)	plant	as above	As above
	Essiac	see Ch.10	formula	Twice a day until 6 weeks after it has cleared.

DISORDERS	THERAPEUTIC PLANTS	PLANT PART USED	FORM USED	METHOD
Cysts	Periwinkle (*Vinca*)	leaf	poultice	Apply poultice per every 24 hours, mixed with comb honey, until cyst breaks.
	Essiac	see Ch.10	formula	Twice a day until 6 weeks after cleared
Varicose Ulcers	Essiac	see Ch.10	formula	As above
	Burdock (*Arctium lappa*)	1st year root	eat as is and decoction	Eat as a vegetable and wash with decoction.
	Cranesbill (*Geranium maculatum*)	plant	infusion	Use as a wash.
	Garlic (*Allium sativum*)	bulb (root)	as is	Eat daily, 3 times, raw in sandwich.
	Ground Ivy (*Nepeta hederacea*)	plant	infusion	Use as a wash.
	Heartsease (*Viola tricolor*)	plant	infusion	Drink and wash with.
	Marigold (*Calendula officinalis*)	flower	ointment	Apply under dry dressing, daily.

DISORDERS	THERAPEUTIC PLANTS	PLANT PART USED	FORM USED	METHOD
Sore Eyes	Bilberry (*Vaccinium myrtillus*)	leaf, before fruiting	infusion	Bathe eyes using dropper to direct wash.
	Eyebright (*Euphrasia officinalis*)	plant	infusion	As above
	Purple Loosestrife (*Lythrum salicaria*)	flowers and leaves	infusion	As above
	Yarrow (*Achillea millefolium*)	plant	infusion	As above
Mouth Ulcers	Sandalwood (*Santalum album*)	heartwood	oil	2 drops in ½ glass warm water, wash.
	Bistort (*Polygonum bistorta*)	plant	decoction	As mouthwash
	Blackberry (*Rubus villosus*)	leaves	infusion	As above
	Sage (*Salvia officinalis*)	plant	oil	3 drops in warm water as wash.

DISORDERS	THERAPEUTIC PLANTS	PLANT PART USED	FORM USED	METHOD
	Wood Sorrel (*Oxalis acetosella*)	fresh leaves	as is	Chew.
	Raspberry (*Rubus idaeus*)	leaf	infusion	As mouth wash.
	Sheep Sorrel (*Rumex acetosella*)	leaf	infusion	As above
	Yarrow (*Achillea millefolium*)	plant	decoction	As above
	Yellow Dock (*Rumex crispus*)	plant	infusion	As above
Peptic Ulcer (Stomach)	Aloe Vera	gel/juice	fresh or commercial	Drink.
	Juniper and Geranium (*Juniperus communis*, *Pelargonium odorantissimum*)		essential oils	2 drops of each in half cup warm water. Drink.
	Carrageen (*sea vegetable*)	plant	decoction	Sweeten and flavour with lemon oil and honey.

DISORDERS	THERAPEUTIC PLANTS	PLANT PART USED	FORM USED	METHOD
	Oats (*Avena sativa*)	grain and stalk	decoction	Drink frequently — also 'flummery' — very runny porridge of oatmeal, strained.
	Marigold (*Calendula officinalis*)	flowers	infusion	Drink frequently.
	Meadowsweet (*Filipendula ulmaria*)	flowers	infusion	Drink frequently.
	Slippery Elm (*Ulmus fulva*)	bark (powdered)	infused or added to soups	Drink with food or alone.
	Violet (*Viola riviniana*)	flowers	infusion	Drink frequently.
	Yarrow (*Achillea millefolium*)	plant	infusion or tincture	Drink in either form, frequently (see dosage in Ch.9).
Facial Herpes	Bogbean (*Menyanthes trifoliata*)	leaves	infusion	Wash frequently in infusion.
Acne	Essiac		formula	Twice a day to clean liver and blood.

DISORDERS	THERAPEUTIC PLANTS	PLANT PART USED	FORM USED	METHOD
	Burdock (*Arctium lappa*)	leaves	decoction	Drink and use as a wash.
		fresh roots	cold infusion	Grate root fine and steep in equal volume of cold water for 24 hours. Squeeze root to extract all water. Take 2 teaspoonfuls each hour up to 10 times a day.
	Garlic (*Allium sativum*)	root	as is	Lots, raw in diet each day.
Warts	Ivy (*Hedera helix*)	leaves	poultice	Pickle leaves in cold apple cider vinegar for 7 days. Use one, folded to fit, strapped on for 24 hours. Repeat daily, for 3 days. Repeat if required. (Pickle keeps indefinitely.)
	Celandine (*Chelidonium majus*)	sap	as is	Apply milky sap direct from stalk to wart.
	Marigold (*Calendula officinalis*)	sap	as is	As above
Colic	Caraway (*Carum carvi*)	seed	infusion	Sip, warm, little and often, till relief.

DISORDERS	THERAPEUTIC PLANTS	PLANT PART USED	FORM USED	METHOD
	Fennel (Foeniculum vulgare)	seed	infusion	As above
	Dill (Anethum graveolens)	seed	infusion	As above
Inflamed wounds	Ox-eye Daisy (Leucanthemum vulgare)	plant	ointment with ghee	Apply liberally. Cover and change once a day, washing with Hydrogen Peroxide between dressings.
Migraine	Feverfew (Chrysanthemum parthenium)	leaves	as is or infusion	Eat or infuse and drink 6 leaves a day to prevent, or as a remedy.
	Blue Flag (Iris versicolor)	root	powdered	Combine one teaspoonful of powder in one cup of infusion.
	Bogbean (Menyanthes trifoliata) or Blue Flag	dried leaves	infusion	
	Bogbean	root	tincture	Combine 1:1 and take 10–20 drops daily.
	Plantain (Plantago lanceolata)	fresh leaves	tincture	
		fresh leaves	crushed	Held on as poultice.

DISORDERS	THERAPEUTIC PLANTS	PLANT PART USED	FORM USED	METHOD
Dry Skin (patches all over)	Lavender (*Lavendula officinalis*)	oil	3 drops in carrier	Sunflower or grapeseed oils as carrier.
	Bogbean (*Menyanthes trifoliata*)	oil	infusion	Drink daily.
	Birch (*Betula pendula*)	dried leaves	in salads	Eat often in season.
	Burdock (*Arctium lappa*)	shoots		
	Chamomile (*Matricaria chamomilla*)	flower		Eat as a salad in season, often;
	Catnip (*Nepeta cataria*)	plant	fresh or dried	or as a soup, or dried, blended and used often as a tea.
	Chickweed (*Stellaria media*)	plant		
	Heartsease (*Viola tricolor*)	flower		
	Meadowsweet (*Filipendula ulmaria*)	flowers		

DISORDERS	THERAPEUTIC PLANTS	PLANT PART USED	FORM USED	METHOD
	Plantain (lance leaf) (*Plantago lanceolata*)	leaf	fresh or dried	Eat as a salad in season, often; or as a soup, or dried, blended and used often as a tea.
	Selfheal (*Prunella vulgaris*)	plant		
Dandruff	Rosemary (*Rosmarinus officinalis*)	leaves or oil	infusion or oil	Infusion, or 4 drops oil in rinsing water. Rub scalp vigorously as rinsing.
Psoriasis on scalp	As above	as above	as above	As above half a cupful cooled with egg yolk added. Use instead of shampoo, rub well, rinse well.
Insomnia, Restless Sleep, Nightmares	Passion flower (*Passiflora incarnata*)	flowers	infusion	Combined as infusion, take nightly for up to no longer than 14 nights.
	Hops (*Humulus lupulus*)	flowers	infusion	
	Valerian (*Valeriana officinalis*)	root (powdered)	with above	Take one cup nightly up to 14 nights.
	Flower essences, e.g. 'Healing Herbs'			Self, or practitioner chosen.

DISORDERS	THERAPEUTIC PLANTS	PLANT PART USED	FORM USED	METHOD
Anaemia	Nasturtium (*Tropaeolum majus*)	leaf, flower or seed	raw or infused	Use in salads or teas. Pickle seeds for winter use.
	Nettle (*Urtica dioica*)	leaf	fresh or dried	Fresh as a vegetable, dried as a tea.
	Watercress (*Nasturtium officinale*)	leaf	fresh	Eat as a vegetable, in salads or soups, or as an infusion/tea.
Psoriasis on Body	Lavender (*Lavandula officinalis*)	flower	oil	4 drops
	Sandalwood (*Santalum album*)	heart wood	oil	8 drops combine with 100 g/4 oz ghee. Use as needed.
	Rose (*Rosa canina*) (and others)	petals	oil	4 drops.
	Wheatgerm	from seed	oil	2 teaspoons.
Rheumatism	Celery (*Apium graveolens*)	seed	infusion	Drink instead of tea or coffee, for weeks or months.
	Heartsease (*Viola tricolor*)	plant	infusion	As above

DISORDERS	THERAPEUTIC PLANTS	PLANT PART USED	FORM USED	METHOD
	Burdock (*Arctium lappa*)	root	grated or oil	Poultice or rub.
	Chickweed (*Stellaria media*)	plant	bath from infusion or tincture	For searing pains. Used over many months restores mobility.
	Nettles (*Urtica dioica*)	young leaves fresh or dry		Eat in season and drink infusion all year.
Hives	Nettle (*Urtica dioica*)	young leaves	oil	Apply liberally.
Septic wounds that won't draw	Periwinkle (*Vinca major or minor*)	leaves	poultice	Change every 24 hours for up to 3 days.
Varicosities Phlebitis Thrombosis Piles (Haemorrhoids)	Yarrow (*Achillea millefolium*)	plant	bath and tincture	Bathe affected area in warm water with 10 drops per 600 ml/1 pt water. Drink 5 drops in a cup of warm water 3 times daily.
	Cocoa (*Theobroma cacao*)	nuts	'butter'	Make a paste with the witch-hazel and cocoa-butter. Apply as needed.
	Witchhazel	tree	infusion	
	Shepherd's Purse (*Capsella bursa-pastoris*)	plant	tincture	Wash — a sitz bath.

DISORDERS	THERAPEUTIC PLANTS	PLANT PART USED	FORM USED	METHOD
	Tormentil (*Potentilla tormentilla*)	root, plant	tincture ⎫	Combine the two tinctures, dilute at 10 drops to 600 ml/1 pt. Use as wash or sitz bath (Note: Eat no red meat).
	Oats (*Avena sativa*)	seed and plant	tincture ⎭	
	Turpentine	tree sap	as is	As above
	Alder (*Alnus serrulata*)	bark	boiled in vinegar	As above
Corns	Ivy (*Hedera helix*)	leaves	in vinegar	Steep leaves covered with apple cider vinegar for 7 days. Apply one folded leaf per corn every 24 hours. Repeat for 3 days.
Verruca	as above	as above	as above	As above
INFECTIONS				
Measles Chickenpox Scarlet fever	Pimpernel (*Pimpernella magna*)	plant	tincture	5–10 drops on cane sugar or honey 3 times a day.
German measles	Yarrow (*Achillea millefolium*)	plant	infusion	Drink frequently.

INFECTIONS	THERAPEUTIC PLANTS	PLANT PART USED	FORM USED	METHOD
Coughs and colds (with or without fever)	Elderflower (*Sambucus nigra*)	flowers	infusion or syrup	As required until relief.
	Elderberry (*Sambucus nigra*)	fruit	as above	
	Rosehip (*Rosa Canina*)	fruit	as above	As above
	Coltsfoot (*Tussilago farfara*)	leaf	as above	As above (see also Jollop formula, pages 80–81).
	Blackberry (*Rubus villosus*)	leaves	infusion or tincture	3 cups infusion per day (½ for children). 4 drops in warm water, hourly.
Diarrhoea	Hawkweed (*Hieracium pilosella*)	plant	decoction	3 cups a day.
	Carrot (*Daucus carota*)	root	soup	
	Cinnamon (*Cinnamomum zeylanicum*)	bark	powdered	One level teaspoonful in 1 cup warm milk.
	Tormentil (*Potentilla tormentilla*)	root	tincture	Combined 1:1, 6 drops in warm water hourly on a fasting stomach.

INFECTIONS	THERAPEUTIC PLANTS	PLANT PART USED	FORM USED	METHOD
	Oat (*Avena sativa*)	plant and seed	tincture	Drink one cup 3 times a day.
	Horsetail (*Equisetum arvense*)	barren stem after fruit	decoction	
Sore throat Tonsillitis	Plantain (*Plantago lanceolata*)	leaves	syrup	Make by alternating layers of leaves (fresh) and cane sugar. Steep for 12 hours, covered. Strain and use. Refrigerate.
	Sandalwood (*Santalum album*)	heartwood	oil	2 drops in half cup of warm water, gargle.
	Pimpernel (*Pimpernella magna*)	root	*cleaned* fresh or dry	Chew it.
	Horseradish (*Cochlearia armoracia*)	root	grated	Apply to outside of throat and keep warm with cloth over and plastic top. One part Horseradish, 2 parts Carrot.
	Carrot (*Daucus carota*)	root	grated	
	Rowan (Mountain ash) (*Sorbus alicuparia*)	fruit, dried	as is	Chew for sore throat or tonsillitis.

INFECTIONS	THERAPEUTIC PLANTS	PLANT PART USED	FORM USED	METHOD
Cystitis	Flax (*Linum usitatissimum*)	seed (linseed)	decoction	One tablespoon per 600 ml/1 pt spring water. Simmer for 10 minutes. Strain, drink as required (real fresh lemon juice can be added if desired).
	Yarrow (*Achillea millefolium*)	plant	tincture	10 drops in one cup of warm water, as needed.
Whooping cough	Ox-eye daisy (*Leucanthemum vulgare*)	plant	infusion fresh or dry	Drink in sips all day. Can be sweetened with honey, if desired.
PARASITES				
Impetigo	Scabious (*Scabiosa columbaria*)	plant	decoction or tincture	Dab on 6 times a day. Use fresh, clean applicator each time. Boil all towels. Apply as poultice to affected area. Change daily, before bed.
	Plantain (*Plantago lanceolata*)	leaf	fresh, crushed	
Scabies	Scabious (*Scabiosa columbaria*)	plant	decoction or tincture	Paint on 3 times a day.
	Rocket (*Hesperia matronalis*)	leaves	as vegetable	Eat lots of this sulphur-rich vegetable when in season.

PARASITES	THERAPEUTIC PLANTS	PLANT PART USED	FORM USED	METHOD
	Flowers of Sulphur (from a pharmacy).	rock powder	ointment	Blended with ghee or lard until stiff. Apply nightly and cover.
Ringworm	Clubmoss (*Lycopodium clavatum*)	plant, dried and powdered	poultice	Make a paste with yogurt and Flowers of Sulphur.
	Scabious (*Scabiosa columbaria*)	plant	decoction or tincture	Apply 3 times a day.
	Celandine (*Chelidonium majus*)	root	tincture	Use tincture to make ointment in animal fat.
	(Note: Gentian Violet, an aniline dye, *always* works for external parasites and fungal infections.)			
Thrush See diet for Candidiasis	Juniper (*Juniperus communis*)	fruit	oil	Apply neat.

PARASITES	THERAPEUTIC PLANTS	PLANT PART USED	FORM USED	METHOD
	Yarrow (*Achillea millefolium*)	plant	infusion or tincture	Drink infusion. Wash area with one teaspoon tincture in half cup warm water.
	Gentian Violet, as above			
Vaginal pruritus (itching)	Scabious (*Scabiosa columbaria*)	plant	bath or compress	
	Blackberry (*Rubus villosus*)	leaves	bath or compress	
Roundworms	Bilberry (*Vaccinium myrtillus*)	leaf	decoction	Drink one cup 3 times a day.
	Garlic (*Allium sativum*)	root, raw	sandwiches	Eat lots of it everyday until worms eliminated.
	Southernwood (*Artemisia abrotanum*)	leaf	infusion or decoction	One cup 3 times a day as needed.
Tapeworm	Castor Oil (*Ricinus communis*)	plant	oil	Fast for 24 hours. Drink 4 tablespoonfuls.
	Walnut oil (*Juglans regia*)	nuts	as above	As above

PARASITES	THERAPEUTIC PLANTS	PLANT PART USED	FORM USED	METHOD
	Tansy (*Tanacetum vulgare*)	seed ⎫	strong infusion	Take one teaspoonful in hot water — one cup before breakfast daily.
	Wormwood (*Artemisia absinthium*)	seed ⎭		
Threadworms	Garlic (*Allium sativum*)	root	raw in sandwiches	Eat plentifully of raw, chopped cloves.
	Lavender (*Lavandula officinalis*)	flower	oil	Three drops in half a cup of hot water before breakfast daily.
	Tansy (*Tanacetum vulgare*)	seed ⎫	strong infusion	One teaspoonful in a cup of hot water before breakfast daily.
	Wormwood (*Artemisia absinthium*)	seed ⎭		
	Silverweed (*Potentilla anserina*)	plant	decoction	One cup daily before breakfast.
Lice and nits	Thyme (*Thymus vulgaris*)	leaf	decoction	As above
	Aloe vera	gel/sap	as is	Rub well into hair. Leave for 30 minutes before washing.

PARASITES	THERAPEUTIC PLANTS	PLANT PART USED	FORM USED	METHOD
	Clove *(Eugenia caryophyllata)*		oil	As above
	Lavender *(Lavandula officinalis)*		oil	Rub well into hair. Leave for 30 minutes before rinsing.
	Eucalyptus *(Eucalyptus globulus)*		oil	As above
	Thyme *(Thymus vulgaris)*		oil	As above
FLY DETERRENT	Tansy *(Tanacetum vulgare)* Elder *(Sambucus nigra)*	dried leaves dried leaves	tied into a bundle	Light end of tightly bound bundle of leaves. Blow out flame and allow to smoulder. Note: Do not leave unattended.
	Peppermint *(Mentha piperata)*	plant, fresh		Hang bundles of fresh mint stalks and leaves in room.
	Sweetpeas	flowers	in a vase	Arrange vases of sweetpeas in room.
FEMALE REPRODUCTION	Raspberry *(Rubus idaeus)*	leaf	infusion	Drink to replace all other drinks during the day. Highly recommended in pregnancy.

FEMALE REPRODUCTION	THERAPEUTIC PLANTS	PLANT PART USED	FORM USED	METHOD
Period pains (to relax and tone muscles)	Yarrow (*Achillea millefolium*)	plant	tincture	Standard dose
Painful periods (Dysmenorrhoes)	Tansy (*Tanacetum vulgare*)	flowers	tincture	As above (Note: Do not take for more than one week).
Pre-Menstrual Tension	Yarrow (*Achillea millefolium*)	plant	infusion	Drink to relieve.
Delayed Periods Painful Periods Bleeding between Periods (Metrorhagia)	} Oats (*Avena sativa*)	seed, plant (straw)	bath	Warm sitz bath for 20 minutes.
To prevent Miscarriage	Raspberry (*Rubus idaeus*)	leaf	infusion	Drink frequently instead of any other drink.
	Vervain (*Verbena officinalis*)	leaf	infusion	As above
Pregnancy (*see page 88*)				

CHAPTER ELEVEN

Case Studies

CASE ONE
ACUTE BRONCHITIS

In 1977, I had a case of a man who had acute bronchitis, with a cough and sore stomach.

REMEDY

To one quart of spring water I added 2 tablespoons linseed. This was simmered for 10 minutes, strained and used to infuse 25 g/1 oz dried Thyme and 25 g/1 oz dried Borage — enough for 2 days. (Can be sweetened with honey, if desired.) The patient sipped the infusion at intervals during the day.

The patient drank one glass of elderflower wine at bedtime and had bone and vegetable broth and lots of real fruit juices. (Do not give squashes or carbonated, artificially flavoured drinks. Also avoid bread, sugar, stodge and dairy products.)

OUTCOME

The patient was back to work in a week, without symptoms.

CASE TWO
RAM WITH ULCERS

This family must have been impressed by the above, because two months later I was asked to treat their ram, to whom the vet had been called on three occasions. Each time he had administered antibiotics for the ulcerous sores on the ram's foreleg. This medication had had no effect, and on the vet's fourth visit he recommended that the ram be sent to the mart and sold. I never saw the animal, but talked about the treatment on the telephone. I knew the man's mother had lots of Vinca minor in her garden and he had Comfrey in his own garden.

The wound began in the foot — not foot-rot. Rose to first joint. Three holes were emitting pussy discharge and refusing to heal. The ram was in a shed, unable to lower his foot to ground and not eating.

REMEDY

Poultice of mashed (raw) Periwinkle (Vinca), leaves and honey was put on the affected area for 24 hours, followed by poultice of fine chopped root of Comfrey and honey. The poultice was changed every 24 hours.

OUTCOME

After a fortnight, the ram was using his leg, the wounds had healed, and he was out grazing again with his ewes.

CASE THREE
COLD SORES

A neighbour, who had three large cold sores (facial herpes) on his lower lip, called. His doctor had prescribed an ointment which was supposed to stop the sores spreading after the first one appeared. This obviously hadn't worked.

REMEDY

I made an infusion of 7 dried Bogbean leaves in half a cup of boiling water. When this was cool, it was applied as a wash. I told him to do this 3 times a day, which he did.

OUTCOME

Within twenty-four hours he could stretch his lip without

soreness and the inflammation had gone down. The scabs cleared in a couple of days.

CASE FOUR
BOILS/SEPTIC SORES

Four years later, our younger daughter came home from a month away with friends. On the front of her left ankle she had a large boil, surrounded by a ring of little satellite boils. On her right foot the nail of the second toe was hanging off and septic where she'd stubbed it on something. She had a nasty looking sore at the edge of her left nostril and several septic sores along the edge of her right ear and under the lobe. She looked a mess!

The friend she'd been staying with had obtained some Marshmallow and Elderflower ointment from a herbalist she'd been using. My daughter was feverish and low-spirited, as well she might be! I washed all the sores with warm saline and put some of the herbalist's ointment on the boil, she took two soluble aspirins and went to bed.

Overnight I worked out a strategy. Her school term began ten days later. I set myself the task of her full recovery by that day. Patently, the blood was below par and her body wasn't cleansing itself properly from the inside. We had to treat both inside and outside.

REMEDY

As the flesh inside her eyelids was red, she didn't appear to be anaemic, but a tonic seemed a good idea anyway. We used a liquid Multivitamin commercial tonic 3 times a day. I also gave her a sandwich of my own bread, with one clove of garlic chopped into it, a teaspoonful of Wheatgerm oil, (vitamin E for the skin) and a teaspoonful of comb honey. She had this sandwich 3 times a day for the next 10 days.

Despite the admonition not to eat raw garlic when also taking homeopathic preparations, I started her on alternating doses of *Silica* 6x (to promote the discharge of pus) and *Calc Flour* 6x (to alleviate the boils). These were Schuessler's Tissue Salts, one or the other every hour, each 6 times a day. I used dilute Hydrogen Peroxide, dribbled and allowed to foam on the septic areas and a poultice of minced Comfrey root (peeled) and comb honey on both the boil and the toe nail. We did this in the morning and again in the evening.

We repeated everything the next day, but a new boil was gathering in her left instep. Poulticed with chopped Vinca and comb honey. Dressed all twice, but left Vinca on for 24 hours.

By the next day, she was more emotionally stable and recovered from her tiring journey home. Repeated everything twice. Her toe was still not responding and the boil in her instep burst after Peroxide wash. I put Vinca on both. The sores in her ears were by then dry and healthy scabs were forming.

Overnight, the inflammation in her instep increased, although the boil was draining. The inflammation was creeping up her foot, making walking impossible. All doses repeated, but changed, alternating Tissue Salts to *Silica* 6x 12 times a day.

The following day, the inflammation in the instep was much reduced and that on the toe was gone. A new eruption on her ear was washed off with Peroxide. In the morning, I put Vinca on instep only; Elder and Marshmallow ointment on the toe; Comfrey ointment on scar of ankle boil. By the evening, all was much improved.

I left the ankle scar without a dressing after a wash. I put Elderflower and Marshmallow ointment on the instep, covered by a dry dressing. My daughter was very brave, as she pulled off the toe nail with sterile forceps. I gave her 2 doses of Rescue Remedy afterwards. By now the ear scars were all dry and the nose sore healed up.

Five days after her return, the inflammation under the instep was almost gone, with a little suppuration overnight. After Peroxide wash, I put on Elderflower and Marshmallow ointment and a waterproof plaster. On the toe I put gauze and the same ointments. She was then able to walk in flip-flops. I only washed the ankle scar — a scab was forming.

In the evening of the same day, I repeated all washes and dressings. She fitted on trainers and walked better.

The next day, we continued with all the doses. The ankle and sole were healing well and dead white skin was sloughing off the sole.

I returned to alternating Silica 6x and Calc Flour 6x on the following day. In the morning, I washed and dressed the toe and sole and in the evening washed but did not dress toe or sole.

On the eighth day, I washed the toe and sole. I used only a small dressing to protect from further infection. There was a new eruption in one of her left ear earring holes and a small one on the inside of her right knee. I washed them and put on ointment as before and plaster.

By the ninth day, all new eruptions had subsided. I used Peroxide washes morning and evening, but no dressings. All doses continued.

My entries for this case history end with the following:

'The difficulty arises now to get a thirteen-year-old

who is much recovered to continue with the internal doses and to refrain from putting earrings of base metal into the half-healed holes!'

OUTCOME

My daughter went back to school as planned on the first day of term completely recovered and had no relapse. I attribute as much of this recovery to the nursing as to the remedies. Washing and dressing wounds is vital on a daily basis.

There are many more case histories in my record book, not all of them involving herbal remedies. They are interesting to read again and show increasing confidence and success as the years have passed. I hope the examples here serve to instil confidence and encouragement in you, if you feel it's time to look for remedies that don't give 'side-effects' and to re-take responsibility for your own well-being.

Helpful Addresses

The Anaphylaxis Campaign
A charity working with United Kingdom NHS allergy specialists to raise awareness of food-induced anaphylaxis.

PO Box 149, Fleet, Hampshire GU13 9XU.
Tel.: 01253 318723.

The Anaphylaxis Campaign in Ireland is a separate organisation that liaises closely with its UK counterpart.
PO Box 4373, Dublin 18, Ireland.

British Association of Dowsers
Secretary, Sycamore Barn, Tamley Lane, Hastingleigh, Ashford, Kent TN25 5HW.

Developer of UKRAIN (herbal based anti-tumour drug)
Dr Jaruslaw Nowicky
Margaretheustrasse 7, 1040 Vienna, Austria.

Five Flower Remedy and Rescue Remedy
Both are available from all well-stocked wholefood shops and homeopathic pharmacies and some other pharmacies. For direct mail orders, contact:

Healing Herbs (Five Flower Remedy)
PO Box 65, Hereford HR2 0UW.

Nelson's Homeopathic Pharmacy (Rescue Remedy)
Available from your nearest wholefood shop or homeopathic pharmacy, or from some ordinary pharmacies.

Suppliers of Seeds, Wild Herbs
John Chambers
15 Westleigh Road, Barton Seagrave, Kettering,
Northants NN15 5AJ.
Tel.: 01536 513748.

Sandro Cafola
Design by Nature
Crettyard, Co. Carlow, Ireland.

Wholesalers for Herbalists
Hambleden Herbs
Court Farm, Milverton, Somerset TA4 1NF.
Tel.: 01823 401205.

The Herbal Apothecary
103 High Street, Syston, Leicester LE7 1GQ.
Tel.: 0116 2602690.

Recommended Reading

Alexandersson, Olof, *Living Water*,
(tr. K. and C. Zweigbergk) Sweden: Gateway Books
1976.

Barnard, Julian and Martina, *The Healing Herbs of Edward Bach*, Hereford: Bach Educational Programme 1988.

Fitter, Fitter and Blamey, *The Wild Flowers of Britain and Northern Europe*, London: Collins 1974.

Gerber, Richard, *Vibrational Medicine*, Santa Fe,
USA: Bear & Co. 1988.

Grieve, Mrs M., *A Modern Herbal*, London: Penguin 1980.

Gurudas, *Flower Essences and Vibrational Healing*, Calif.,
USA: Cassandra Press 1983.

Hanh, Thich Nhat, *Peace is Every Step*, London:
Rider 1991.

Holmes, Peter, *The Energetics of Western Herbs*,
Boulder, Calif., USA: Artemis Press 1989.

Irish Red Cross Society and The Order of Malta, *First Aid Manual*, Dublin: Irish Red Cross Society 1990.

Kloss, Jethro, *Back to Eden*, Calif., USA:
Woodbridge Press 1939.

Lust, John, *The Herb Book*, London: Bantam Books 1974.

Mességué, Maurice, *Health Secrets of Plants and Herbs*,
London: Pan Books 1981.

Ni, Maoshing, *The Yellow Emperor's Classic of Medicine*,
Boston, Mass: Shambhala 1995.

Peat, F. David, *Blackfoot Physics*,
London: Fourth Estate 1995.

Scallan, Christine, *Irish Herbal Cures*,
Dublin: Gill & Macmillan 1994.

Singhal, G. D. and Patterson, T. J. S, *Synopsis of Ayurveda*,
Delhi: Oxford University Press 1993.

Siegel, Bernie, *Peace, Love and Health*, London: Rider 1990.

Siegel, Bernie, *Living, Loving and Healing*, London: Aquarian Press 1993.

Treben, Maria, *Health Through God's Pharmacy*, (22nd edition) Austria: Ennsthaler 1994.

Tsu, Lao, *Tao Te Ching*, (tr. Gia-fu Feng and Jane English) Aldershot: Wildwood House 1973.

Vogel, Dr H. C. A., *The Nature Doctor*, (50th edition) Edinburgh: Mainstream Publishing 1989.

Weed, Susun S., *Healing Wise*, New York: Ash Tree Publishing 1989.

Weed, Susun S., *Menopausal Years The Wise Woman Way*, New York: Ash Tree Publishing 1992.

Westwood, Christine, *Aromatherapy A Guide for Home Use*, Dorset: Amberwood Publishing 1991.

Wright, Machaelle Small, *MAP — Medical Assistance Programme*, Virginia, USA: Jefferson 1994.

Zysk, Kenneth G., *Ascetism and Healing in Ancient India*, Delhi: Oxford University Press 1991.

Index